Pediatric Ophthalmology
AND **Strabismus**

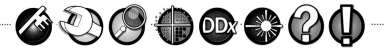

Rapid Diagnosis in Ophthalmology
Series Editors: Jay S. Duker MD, *Marian S. Macsai* MD
Associate Editor: Gary S. Schwartz MD

Anterior Segment
Bruno Machado Fontes, Marian S. Macsai
ISBN 978-0-323-04406-6

Lens and Glaucoma
Joel S. Schuman, Viki Christopoulos, Deepinder K. Dhaliwal,
Malik Y. Kahook, Robert J. Noecker
ISBN 978-0-323-04443-1

Neuro-ophthalmology
Jonathan D. Trobe
ISBN 978-0-323-04456-1

Oculoplastic and Reconstructive Surgery
Jeffrey A. Nerad, Keith D. Carter, Mark Alford
ISBN 978-0-323-05386-0

Pediatric Ophthalmology and Strabismus
Mitchell B. Strominger
ISBN 978-0-323-05168-2

Retina
Adam H. Rogers, Jay S. Duker
ISBN 978-0-323-04959-7

Commissioning Editors: Russell Gabbedy, Belinda Kuhn
Development Editor: Martin Mellor Publishing Services Ltd
Project Manager: Rory MacDonald
Design Manager: Stewart Larking
Illustration Manager: Merlyn Harvey
Illustrator: Jennifer Rose
Marketing Manager(s) (UK/USA): John Canelon/Lisa Damico

Series Editors: Jay S. **Duker** MD, Marian S. **Macsai** MD
Associate Editor: Gary S. **Schwartz** MD

Rapid Diagnosis in Ophthalmology
Pediatric
Ophthalmology
AND
Strabismus

By
Mitchell B. Strominger MD,
Chief, Pediatric Ophthalmology and Ocular Motility; Associate Professor of
Ophthalmology and Pediatrics, TUFTS-New England Medical Center, Boston,
MA, USA

Series Editors
Jay S. Duker MD,
Director, New England Eye Center, Vitreoretinal Diseases and Surgery Service;
Professor and Chair of Ophthalmology, Tufts University School of Medicine,
Boston, MA, USA

Marian S. Macsai MD,
Chief, Division of Ophthalmology, Evanston Northwestern Healthcare; Professor
and Vice-Chair, Department of Ophthalmology, Feinberg School of Medicine,
Northwestern University, Chicago, IL, USA

Associate Editor
Gary S. Schwartz MD,
Adjunct Associate Professor, Department of Ophthalmology, University of
Minnesota, Minneapolis, MN, USA

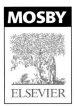

MOSBY

ELSEVIER

MOSBY
ELSEVIER

Mosby is an affiliate of Elsevier Inc.

© 2008, Elsevier Inc. All rights reserved.

First published 2008

The following figures are from Taylor D, Hoyt CS (Eds) 2005 Pediatric Ophthalmology and Strabismus, 3rd edn. Saunders, London: Figures 20.2B, 22.11–22.13, 22.17, 22.20, 22.26, 30.7, 39.3, 39.5, 39.6, 39.9, 44.6–44.8, 45.4, 45.5, 46.1, 47.11A,C, 48.1, 48.2, 50.2A,D, 50.5A, 50.6A, 51.6, 51.8, 51.10, 51.22, 52.6, 52.7, 59.14, 65.2, 65.9, 68.6, 68.15, 73.18, 74.1, 74.2, 80.2, 80.3, 82.5, 84.4, 85.1, and 85.2 and Tables 51.1, 65.1, and 65.2.

The following figure is from Spalton D et al. 2005 Atlas of Clinical Ophthalmology, 3rd edn. Mosby, London: Figure 9.10.

ISBN 978-0-323-05168-2

British Library Cataloguing in Publication Data
A catalogue record for this book is available from the British Library

Library of Congress Cataloging in Publication Data
A catalog record for this book is available from the Library of Congress

Notice
Medical knowledge is constantly changing. Standard safety precautions must be followed, but as new research and clinical experience broaden our knowledge, changes in treatment and drug therapy may become necessary or appropriate. Readers are advised to check the most current product information provided by the manufacturer of each drug to be administered to verify the recommended dose, the method and duration of administration, and contraindications. It is the responsibility of the practitioner, relying on experience and knowledge of the patient, to determine dosages and the best treatment for each individual patient. Neither the Publisher nor the author assumes any liability for any injury and/or damage to persons or property arising from this publication.

The Publisher

ELSEVIER your source for books, journals and multimedia in the health sciences

www.elsevierhealth.com

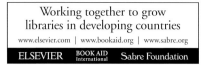

Working together to grow
libraries in developing countries

www.elsevier.com | www.bookaid.org | www.sabre.org

ELSEVIER   BOOK AID International   Sabre Foundation

The publisher's policy is to use **paper manufactured from sustainable forests**

Printed in China
Last digit is the print number: 9   8   7   6   5   4   3   2   1

Contents

Contents

13 Strabismus: Miscellaneous

14 Strabismus: Nystagmus

Contents

Given the complexity and quantity of clinical knowledge required to correctly identify and treat ocular disease, a quick reference text with high quality color images represents an invaluable resource to the busy clinician. Despite the availability of extensive resources online to clinicians, accessing these resources can be time consuming and often requires filtering through unnecessary information. In the exam room, facing a patient with an unfamiliar presentation or complicated medical problem, this series will be an invaluable resource.

This handy pocket sized reference series puts the knowledge of world-renowned experts at your fingertips. The standardized format provides the key element of each disease entity as your first encounter. The additional information on the clinical presentation, ancillary testing, differential diagnosis and treatment, including the prognosis, allows the clinician to instantly diagnose and treat the most common diseases seen in a busy practice. Inclusion of classical clinical color photos provides additional assurance in securing an accurate diagnosis and initiating management.

Regardless of the area of the world in which the clinician practices, these handy references guides will provide the necessary resources to both diagnose and treat a wide variety of ophthalmic diseases in all ophthalmologic specialties. The clinician who does not have easy access to sub-specialists in Anterior Segment, Glaucoma, Pediatric Ophthalmology, Strabismus, Neuro-ophthalmology, Retina, Oculoplastic and Reconstructive Surgery, and Uveitis will find these texts provide an excellent substitute. World-wide recognized experts equip the clinician with the elements needed to accurately diagnose treat and manage these complicated diseases, with confidence aided by the excellent color photos and knowledge of the prognosis.

The field of knowledge continues to expand for both the clinician in training and in practice. As a result we find it a challenge to stay up to date in the diagnosis and management of every disease entity that we face in a busy clinical practice. This series is written by an international group of experts who provide a clear, structured format with excellent photos.

It is our hope that with the aid of these six volumes, the clinician will be better equipped to diagnose and treat the diseases that affect their patients, and improve their lives.

Marian S. Macsai and Jay S. Duker

Preface

The examination of children in a busy ophthalmic practice can be a daunting task. A child's attention span is short and the examination needs to be quick and directed. Once a diagnosis is suspected further testing and treatment needs to be initiated. Discussions about the diagnosis, treatment and prognosis then must take place quickly with the child's guardian prior to complete distraction from the patient.

A quick reference text such this provides the busy clinician key points about pediatric ophthalmic and strabismic diagnosis that can streamline the examination of the child. It also provides essential information that can be used in discussions with the guardian about treatment and prognosis in a timely fashion.

Mitchell B. Strominger

I am grateful for the generosity of the authors and editors of Taylor D, Hoyt CS, Pediatric Ophthalmology and Strabismus (2005) to allow use of figures from their work.

To my mentor, Norman Medow, MD, who has provided me opportunity, knowledge, guidance, and friendship over these many years. Also to my wife Jaclyn who is always loving and supportive; and my daughter Sydney whose afternoon weekend naps during her first year of life provided me the quiet time to write.

Mitchell B. Strominger

Acknowledgments/Dedication

Section 1

Pediatric: Amblyopia

Strabismic Amblyopia

Key Facts

- Visual impairment without apparent structural pathology (amblyopia) developing in a consistently deviating eye
- Cortical suppression of image from deviating eye secondary to competitive inhibition in order to prevent diplopia and visual confusion
- Grating acuity is worse than in other forms of amblyopia

Clinical Findings

- Ocular misalignment
- Reduced visual acuity in deviated eye

Ancillary Testing

- Full ophthalmic examination to rule out structural lesion as cause of deprivational strabismus
- Consider neuroimaging if optic nerve or visual pathway dysfunction
- Sensory motor testing
- Motility testing to rule out restrictive strabismus or cranial neuropathy
- Full cycloplegic retinoscopy and manifest refraction

Differential Diagnosis

- Anisometropic amblyopia
- Isometropic amblyopia
- Deprivational amblyopia

Treatment

- Fully correct refractive error in both eyes
- Treat underlying amblyopia with patching or atropine 1% penalization to good seeing eye
  - Begin patching 2 h/day and increase frequency if not responding
- Surgically correct strabismus

Prognosis

- **Depends on:**
  - age of detection • compliance with treatment
- Worse prognosis in children over age 8
- Dismal prognosis in adults

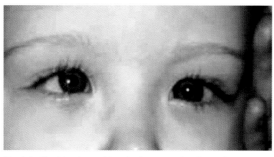

Fig. 1.1 Strabismic amblyopia from esotropia and hypertropia.

Anisometropic Amblyopia

Key Facts

- Difference in refractive error between (both) eyes, leading to visual impairment in one eye without apparent structural pathology (amblyopia) if not corrected early
- Typically asymptomatic and detected only with visual acuity testing or screening
- Age range of detection usually 3–7 years
- Association with strabismus hastens diagnosis
- **More common with:**
  - anisometropic hyperopia • astigmatism • high myopia
- Less common with anisometropic myopia because of using myopic eye for near viewing

Clinical Findings

- Visual acuity typically ranges from 20/40 to 20/80 (moderate) and 20/100 to 20/400 (severe) in amblyopic eye, with intraocular difference of greater than three lines of vision
- Can occur with hyperopic difference of >0.5 D of spherical equivalent but typically greater
- Can occur with astigmatic difference of >1.5 D in any meridian but typically greater
- Can occur with myopic difference of >2.0 D but typically greater
- Otherwise normal ocular examination

Ancillary Testing

- Complete ophthalmic examination to rule out structural abnormality
- Full cycloplegic retinoscopy and manifest refraction
- Sensory motor testing

Differential Diagnosis

- Strabismic amblyopia
- Isometropic amblyopia
- Deprivational amblyopia

Treatment

- Fully correct refractive error in both eyes
- If full refractive error not prescribed, maintain anisometropia
- Treat underlying amblyopia with patching or atropine 1% penalization to good seeing eye
  - If after 2 months of wearing the optical correction the visual acuity has not equalized, begin patching 2 h/day and increase frequency if not responding
- Consider contact lenses in older children to reduce aniseikonia
- Refractive surgery may be considered but is currently being studied in patients who do not tolerate a contact lens and have a high amount of anisometropia

Prognosis

- **Depends on:**
  - age of detection • compliance with wearing optical correction and treatment of residual amblyopia
- Up to 96% of patients aged 3–7 years will improve two or more lines of visual acuity with treatment
- Possible 27% improvement of two or more lines of visual acuity in patients aged 10–18 years with treatment
- Poor prognosis in adults

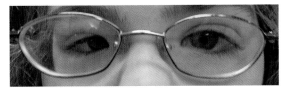

Fig. 1.2 Amblyopia of the right eye from anisometropic myopia.

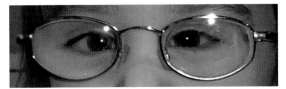

Fig. 1.3 Amblyopia of the right eye from anisometropic hyperopia.

Isometropic (Ametropic) Amblyopia

Key Facts

- Visual impairment without apparent structural pathology (amblyopia) secondary to large bilateral refractive errors
- Typically asymptomatic and detected only with visual acuity testing or screening
- Age range of detection usually 3–7 years
- Association with strabismus is rare

Clinical Findings

- **Visual acuity typically ranges from 20/40 to 20/80 (moderate):**
  - bilateral hyperopia of >5 D or
  - bilateral astigmatism of >2.5 D in any meridian or
  - bilateral myopia of >8 D
  - otherwise normal ocular examination

Ancillary Testing

- Complete ophthalmic examination to rule out structural abnormality
- Full cycloplegic retinoscopy and manifest refraction
- Sensory motor testing

Differential Diagnosis

- Strabismic amblyopia
- Anisometropic amblyopia
- Deprivational amblyopia

Treatment

- Fully correct refractive error in both eyes with glasses as determined with cycloplegic retinoscopy
- In high hyperopia, as long as aniometropia is maintained and no strabismus is present the amount of correction can be reduced by 1–2 D to allow for accommodation
- Consider contact lenses in older children

Prognosis

- Visual acuity improves slowly with treatment
- Visual acuity may not improve to better than 20/25 to 20/40

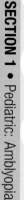

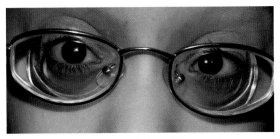

Fig. 1.4 Isometropic amblyopia from high myopia.

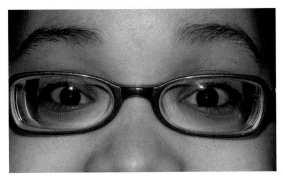

Fig. 1.5 Similar patient as in above figure. Isometropic amblyopia from bilateral high myopia.

Deprivation Amblyopia

Key Facts

- Amblyopia caused by structural abnormality that occludes visual axis or prevents clear foveal image
- Typically asymptomatic and detected only with visual acuity testing or screening
- Age range of detection usually 3–7 years
- Association with strabismus hastens diagnosis

Clinical Findings

- Visual acuity ranges from 20/40 to 20/80 (moderate) and 20/100 to 20/400 (severe) despite treatment of underlying structural cause
- **Common causes include:**
  - ptosis • other asymmetric lid abnormalities • corneal opacity • hyphema • cataract • vitreous hemorrhage
- Possible occlusion amblyopia secondary to over-aggressive patching in treatment of other forms of amblyopia

Ancillary Testing

- Complete ophthalmic examination to determine structural abnormality
- Full cycloplegic retinoscopy and manifest refraction

Differential Diagnosis

- Strabismic amblyopia
- Isometropic amblyopia
- Anisometropic amblyopia

Treatment

- Treat primary cause of deprivation amblyopia
- Treat underlying amblyopia with patching or atropine 1% penalization to good seeing eye
  - Begin patching 2 h/day and increase frequency if not responding

Prognosis

- **Depends on:**
  - age of detection • cause of structural abnormality • compliance with treatment

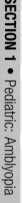

SECTION 1 • Pediatric: Amblyopia

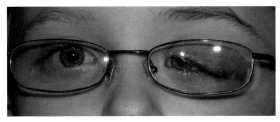

Fig. 1.6 Deprivation amblyopia from left upper lid plexiform neurofibroma.

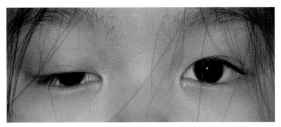

Fig. 1.7 Deprivation amblyopia from right upper lid ptosis.

Section 2
Pediatric: Infectious

TORCHES

Key Facts

- Congenital or delayed reactivation of ocular disease, maternally transmitted, resulting in direct infection or teratogenic effect
- **TORCHES:** toxoplasmosis, rubella, cytomegalic inclusion disease, herpesviruses (including Epstein–Bar), and syphilis
- **Toxoplasmosis:**
  - obligate intracellular organism *Toxoplasma gondii* • cats are definitive host— oocysts reside in intestine then are secreted fecally and ingested by humans • oocysts have predilection for retina and can remain dormant indefinitely or rupture • acquired congenitally via transplacental transmission or in childhood
- **Rubella (German measles):**
  - transplacental transmission of rubella virus • eye (cataracts, pigmentary retinopathy), ear (deafness), and cardiac abnormalities in association with microcephaly
- **Cytomegalovirus:**
  - transplacential transmission, contact via infected birth canal, or infected breast milk • herpesvirus family • acquired infections occur in the immunocompromised • deafness, microcephaly, periventricular calcifications, hematologic and hepatic abnormalities
- **Herpes simplex virus (HSV):**
  - congenital infection occurs during passage through infected birth canal • acquired infections (HSV type 1 affects skin, eyes, and mouth; HSV type 2 is a venereal infection acquired via genital contact) • most neonatal cases are disseminated and involve the central nervous system, lungs, liver, and adrenal glands • minority of cases cause skin lesions, mouth sores, and keratoconjunctivitis
- **Syphilis:**
  - spirochete *Treponema pallidum* • higher rate of transmission in late untreated maternal infection • prematurity in association with hepatosplenopmegaly, pneumonia, jaundice, anemia, and lymphadenopathy • periostosis or metaphysicial abnormalities on x-ray • Hutchinson triad (wide peg-shaped teeth, eighth nerve deafness, interstitial keratitis)

Clinical Findings

- **Toxoplasmosis:**
  - retinitis with possible choroiditis or anterior uveitis • reactivation may occur adjacent to an old scar (satellite lesion) • intracranial calcifications, hepatosplenomegaly, microcephaly, and developmental delay
- **Rubella:**
  - nuclear (morgagnian) cataract • microphthalmos • salt and pepper or pseudo retinitis pigmentosa retinopathy
- **Cytomegalovirus:**
  - microphthalmia, cataracts, uveitis, and retinochoroiditis • diffuse retinal necrosis with whitening, hemorrhage, and venous sheathing
- **Herpes simplex:**
  - conjunctivitis, keratitis (epithelial or stromal), cataracts, and retinochoroiditis
- **Syphilis:**
  - salt and pepper or pseudo retinitis pigmentosa retinopathy • anterior uveitis or glaucoma • bilateral interstitial keratitis

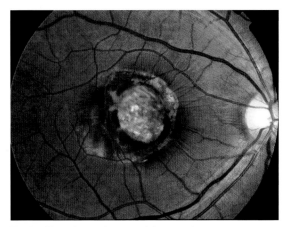

Fig. 2.1 Toxoplasmosis scar, right macula.

TORCHES (Continued)

Ancillary Testing

- **Toxoplasmosis:**
  - ELISA (enzyme-linked immunoassay) • because IgM does not cross the placenta, positivity in the infant is evidence for congenital infection
- **Rubella:**
  - serologic testing • isolation of virus from lens material or pharyngeal swabs
- **Cytomegalovirus:**
  - serologic testing • isolation of virus from secretions
- **Herpes simplex:**
  - viral cultures • PCR
- **Syphilis:**
  - VDRL • Fluorescent treponemal antibody absorption or microhemagglutination assay for *T. pallidum* antibodies • Long bone x-rays

Differential Diagnosis

- Toxoplasmosis, rubella, cytomegalic inclusion disease, herpesviruses (including Epstein–Bar), and syphilis (TORCHES)
- Other intrauterine infections

Treatment

- **Toxoplasmosis:**
  - treated primarily if vision-threatening, because active lesions become quiescent after 1–2 months • systemic corticosteroids in association with pyrimethamine and sulfadiazine plus folinic acid, or clindamycin, or trimethoprim–sulfamethoxazole
- **Rubella:**
  - cataract extraction—beware of excess postoperative inflammation
- **Cytomegalovirus:**
  - intravenous and intravitreal ganciclovir • oral valacyclovir in non–vision-threatening cases
- **Herpes simplex:**
  - oral acyclovir • topical (trifluridine 1% one drop nine times per day, vidarabine 3% ointment five times per day; deep stromal or disciform may require topical corticosteroids) • intravenous antivirals in disseminated disease
- **Syphilis:**
  - intravenous aqueous penicillin G

Prognosis

- **Toxoplasmosis:**
  - if lesion involves macula or optic nerve, vision can be permanently affected
- **Rubella:**
  - depends on extent of retinopathy, density of cataract, and degree of microcephaly
- **Cytomegalovirus:**
  - depends on extent of retinopathy and whether macula or optic nerve involved
- **Herpes simplex:**
  - depends on extent of disseminated disease and location of corneal infection
- **Syphilis:**
  - depends on extent of congenital abnormalities versus active treatable disease

DDx

SECTION 2 • Pediatric: Infectious

14

Ophthalmia Neonatorum

Key Facts

- Conjunctivitis affecting newborns during first month of life
- Transmitted to newborn when passing through birth canal in cases of *Neisseria gonorrhoeae* and *Chlamydia trachomatis*
- Within first few days after birth suggests toxic reaction to silver nitrate prophylaxis
- Within 2–5 days after birth, typically due to *N. gonorrhoeae*
- Within 5–14 days after birth, typically due to *C. trachomatis*
- Could also be caused by *Staphylococcus aureus*, *Streptococcus pneumoniae*, and *Haemophilus*

Clinical Findings

- Hyperacute papillary reaction
- Mild conjunctival injection if secondary to silver nitrate
- Serosanguineous discharge that progresses to thick purulent discharge with chemosis and eyelid edema if secondary to *N. gonorrhoeae*
- Mild mucopurulent discharge with mild chemosis and lid swelling if secondary to *C. trachomatis*

Ancillary Testing

- Evaluate mother for infection
- Routine gram stain and cultures for *Staph. aureus*, *Strep. pneumoniae*, and *Haemophilus*
- **N. gonorrhoeae**:
  - conjunctival cultures • gram stain (gram-negative diplococci)
- **C. trachomatis**:
  - conjunctival culture with chlamydial transport medium • Giemsa stain (basophilic intracytoplasmic inclusion bodies) • PCR and direct immunofluorescent monoclonal antibody stain • chest x-ray for possible chlamydial pneumonitis

Differential Diagnosis

- Chemical conjunctivitis
- *N. gonorrhoeae* conjunctivitis
- *C. trachomatis* conjunctivitis
- *Staph. aureus*, *Strep. pneumoniae*, and *Haemophilus* conjunctivitis
- Herpes simplex conjunctivitis
- Nasolacrimal duct obstruction

Treatment

- **N. gonorrhoeae conjunctivitis**:
  - intravenous ceftriaxone • ocular saline irrigation • supplemental topical antibiotics
- **C. trachomatis conjunctivitis**:
  - oral erythromycin, 50 mg/kg per day, in four divided doses for 14 days
  - topical 0.5% erythromycin ointment four times per day • must also treat mother and father

Prognosis

- Excellent if treated in timely and appropriate fashion
- *N. gonorrhoeae* can invade intact corneal epithelium and cause keratitis, corneal ulceration, and perforation
- *C. trachomatis* can cause tarsal conjunctival scarring and corneal micropannus

Bacterial Conjunctivitis

Key Facts

- Most common ocular infection in children
- Peak incidence at 1–3 years of age
- **Most common organisms:**
  - *Haemophilus influenzae* • *Streptococcus pneumoniae* • *Staphylococcus aureus* • *Moraxella*
- Association with concurrent otitis and/or sinusitis

Clinical Findings

- Purulent green or yellow discharge
- Hyperemia of bulbar conjunctiva
- Matting (crusting) of lashes

Ancillary Testing

- Conjunctival gram stain and culture
- Fluorescein staining to rule out keratoconjunctivitis (e.g. herpes)

Differential Diagnosis

- Viral conjunctivitis
- Allergic conjunctivitis
- Herpes simplex conjunctivitis
- Nasolacrimal duct obstruction

Treatment

- Broad-spectrum topical bacteriocidal antibiotic drop preferred (e.g. moxifloxicin t.i.d. for 5 days)
- Lid hygiene

Prognosis

- Excellent prognosis if treated in timely and appropriate fashion
- If placed on a bacteriocidal antibiotic (e.g. moxifloxicin), the time to eradicate 99.9% of the bacteria with in vitro models is within hours
  - This allows for early return to school or day care without significant risk of spread

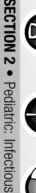

SECTION 2 • Pediatric: Infectious

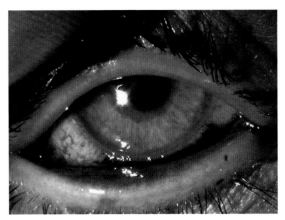

Fig. 2.2 Hyperacute: *N. meningitides* conjunctivitis with a central corneal epithelial erosion. (Courtesy of Seema Verma.)

Viral Conjunctivitis

Key Facts

- Ocular discomfort, photophobia, and tearing
- Most common causes are adenovirus or herpes simplex virus (HSV)
- Spread is via droplet or person to person contact
- **Epidemic keratoconjunctivitis:**
  - adenovirus serotypes 8, 11, and 19 • subepithelial gray-white infiltrates in later stage • usually resolves in 14–21 days
- **Pharyngeal conjunctival fever:**
  - adenovirus serotypes 3, 4, and 7 • pharyngitis and fever
- **HSV:**
  - typically associated with vesicular dermatitis • corneal dendritic ulceration
- Acute hemorrhagic conjunctivitis (enterovirus, coxsackievirus)

Clinical Findings

- Acute follicular conjunctivitis
- Conjunctival injection and chemosis
- Watery discharge
- Membranes and pseudomembranes possible
- Lid edema
- Preauricular adenopathy
- **Epidemic keratoconjunctivitis:**
  - corneal subepithelial infiltrates
- **HSV:**
  - corneal punctuate epithelial stain • dendritic ulceration • vesicular dermatitis

Ancillary Testing

- Viral cultures typically not required
- Fluorescein staining to rule out corneal epithelial pathology or dendrite

Differential Diagnosis

- Bacterial conjunctivitis
- Allergic conjunctivitis
- Nasolacrimal duct obstruction
- Preseptal or orbital cellulitis

Treatment

- Epidemic keratoconjunctivitis or pharyngeal conjunctival fever
  - Primarily palliative (cool compress, ocular lubricants) • Topical corticosteroids can be considered for severe membrane formation or significant visual acuity reduction secondary to subepithelial infiltrates (controversial because corticosteroids can prolong duration of subepithelial infiltrates, and to prevent recurrence, need to be tapered over weeks to months)
- **HSV:**
  - topical antivirals (3% vidarabine ointment five times a day or 1% trifluridine drops nine times per day) • cool compress • topical antibiotic to dermatitis to prevent bacterial superinfection

Prognosis

- Usually excellent but conjunctival scarring and symblepharon can occur
- Can have recurrence with HSV
- Topical corticosteroids can cause glaucoma in steroid responders and cataract formation, and may prolong course of subepithelial infiltrates
- May be infectious for up to 1 week

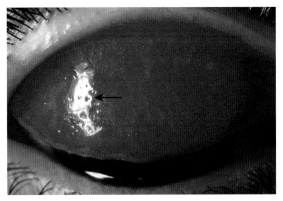

Fig. 2.3 Acute follicular adenovirus conjunctivitis. Small follicles (arrow) surrounded by infiltrated and hyperemic conjunctiva. (From Taylor D, Hoyt CS 2005 Pediatric Ophthalmology and Strabismus, 3rd edn. Saunders, London.)

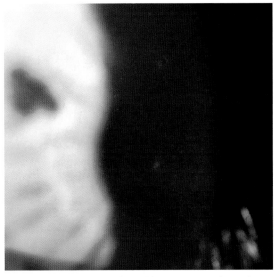

Fig. 2.4 Epithelial infiltrate from the same case shown in Fig. 2.3. (From Taylor D, Hoyt CS 2005 Pediatric Ophthalmology and Strabismus, 3rd edn. Saunders, London.)

Preseptal Cellulitis

Key Facts

- Periorbital lid edema and erythema secondary to infection or inflammation of tissues anterior to orbital septum
- **Most likely infectious organisms include:**
  - *Staphylococcus* • *Streptococcus* • *Haemophilus*
- Commonly associated with upper respiratory tract infection or sinusitis but can be secondary to trauma or localized skin infection

Clinical Findings

- Eyelid and possible periorbital erythema and edema
- Conjunctival injection and chemosis may be present
- Normal vision, extraocular motility, and optic nerve function
- No proptosis or pain on eye movements

Ancillary Testing

- If conjunctivitis present, consider culture
- Consider white blood cell count and blood cultures if febrile
- Watch for progression to orbital cellulitis

Differential Diagnosis

- Chalazion
- Eyelid tumor
- Orbital cellulitis

Treatment

- Oral or systemic broad-spectum antibiotics depending on severity of infection

Prognosis

- Usually excellent if treated appropriately and in timely fashion

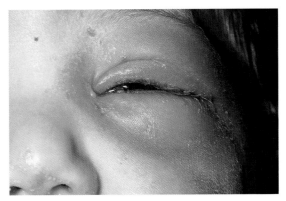

Fig. 2.5 Preseptal cellulitis due to *Haemophilus influenzae* in a 6-month-old infant. (From Taylor D, Hoyt CS 2005 Pediatric Ophthalmology and Strabismus, 3rd edn. Saunders, London.)

Orbital Cellulitis

Key Facts

- Infection or inflammation of tissues posterior to orbital septum
- Most likely infectious organisms include *Staphylococcus*, *Streptococcus*, and *Haemophilus*, except in immunocompromised patients, who can develop fungal and gram-negative infections
- Commonly spreads from associated sinusitis
- Vision loss and diplopia may be present

Clinical Findings

- Ocular pain
- Eyelid erythema and edema
- Conjunctival chemosis
- Restricted extraocular motility with possible proptosis
- Possible optic nerve involvement with reduced visual acuity
- Disease complications may include cavernous sinus thrombosis and meningitis
- Fever more likely than in preseptal cellulitis

Ancillary Testing

- Full ophthalmic examination including extraocular motility, pupil and color testing
- CT or MRI scan of orbits and sinuses to evaluate sinusitis and subperiosteal abscess
- Culture sinus drainage if present
- White blood cell count and blood cultures if febrile

Differential Diagnosis

- **Orbital tumor, including:**
  - rhabdomyosarcoma • lymphangioma • leukemia
- Orbital pseudotumor
- Preseptal cellulitis

Treatment

- Broad-spectrum intravenous antibiotics
- Possible, by otolaryngologist, drainage of involved sinuses
- Drainage of subperiostial abscess may be required if no response to treatment

Prognosis

- Usually excellent if treated appropriately and in timely fashion

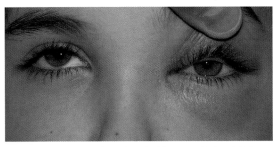

Fig. 2.6 Proptosis and conjunctival hyperemia in orbital cellulitis.

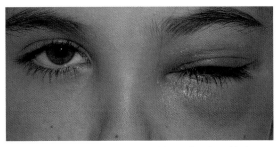

Fig. 2.7 Periobital hyperemia and lid swelling in orbital cellulitis.

Section 3
Pediatric: Inflammatory

Allergic Conjunctivitis

Key Facts

- **Common key facts:**
  - type 1 hypersensitivity reaction (seasonal, vernal, and atopic)
  - type 4 delayed-type cell-mediated hypersensitivity reaction (vernal and atopic)
  - symptoms include itching and conjunctival inflammation
  - association with asthma, allergic rhinitis, and atopic dermatitis
- **Seasonal allergic conjunctivitis:**
  - common in children
  - occurs in spring and fall in association with such airborne allergens as grasses, flowers, weeds, and trees
  - perennial allergic condition secondary to dust mites or pet dander
- **Vernal conjunctivitis:**
  - additional type 4 hypersensitivity reaction (cell-mediated)
  - usually occurs in spring and fall
  - most patients <10 years old
  - most commonly affecting boys until after puberty, when equal between males and females
  - seasonal exacerbations can occur
  - photophobia and intense itching
  - palpebral form with giant cobblestone papillae
  - limbal form with Horner–Trantas dots most marked superiorly (discrete nodules with vascular core, white center filled with eosinophils)
  - cornea epithelial defect (shield ulcer)
- **Atopic conjunctivitis:**
  - type 1 and cell-mediated immunity
  - rare in children
  - occurs in male teenagers
  - occurs in patients with atopic dermatitis, eczema, and asthma
  - morning mucus discharge

Clinical Findings

- **Seasonal allergic conjunctivitis:**
  - chemosis
  - lower lid ecchymosis (allergic shiner)
  - conjunctival follicular reaction
- **Vernal conjunctivitis:**
  - giant papillae, nodules with blood vessels
  - upper eyelid tarsal conjunctiva preferentially affected
  - thick ropy discharge
  - limbal form with Horner–Trantas dots
  - superior corneal micropannus
  - punctuate epithelial erosions that can progress to epithelial defect (shield ulcer)
- **Atopic conjunctivitis:**
  - inferior palpebral conjunctival papillae
  - eyelid dermatitis
  - lateral canthal ulceration
  - severe disease can lead to keratoconus, lichenified eyelids with ectropion and lagophthalmos, and conjunctival subepithelial fibrosis

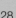

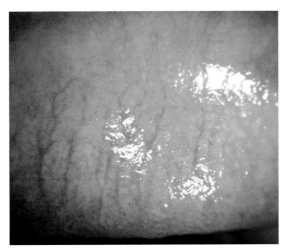

Fig. 3.1 Upper tarsal conjunctival infiltrate in seasonal allergic conjunctivitis. Note the hazy views of the tarsal blood vessels due to the thickened conjunctiva, and the very small papillae in the specular reflex. (From Taylor D, Hoyt CS 2005 Pediatric Ophthalmology and Strabismus, 3rd edn. Saunders, London.)

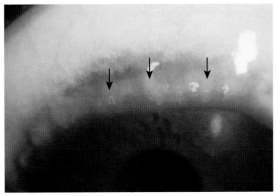

Fig. 3.2 Trantas dots in limbal vernal keratoconjunctivitis. These are very small pale dots at the apices of the papillae (arrows). (From Taylor D, Hoyt CS 2005 Pediatric Ophthalmology and Strabismus, 3rd edn. Saunders, London.)

Ancillary Testing
- **Common ancillary testing:**
  - allergy testing for offending agent
- **Seasonal allergic conjunctivitis:**
  - conjunctival scrapings show eosinophils
- **Vernal conjunctivitis:**
  - conjunctival scrapings show mast cell or lymphocyte-mediated response
  - conjunctival biopsy shows substantia propria infiltrated with lymphocytes, plasma cells, and eosinophils
- **Atopic conjunctivitis:**
  - dermatologic examination

Differential Diagnosis
- Bacterial conjunctivitis
- Chemical conjunctivitis
- Viral conjunctivitis
- Giant papillary conjunctivitis

Treatment
- **Common treatments:**
  - remove from environment offending allergen
  - oral antihistamines less effective and have side effects (e.g. sedation)
  - topical H_1-blocking antihistamines and mast cell stabilizers
  - topical corticosteroids—monitor closely for side effects, including glaucoma and cataracts

Prognosis
- Excellent if adequate therapy begun early
  - Sometimes medications need to be started just before onset of seasonal allergen as prophylaxis

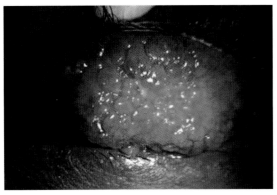

Fig. 3.3 Giant papillae in vernal keratoconjunctivitis.

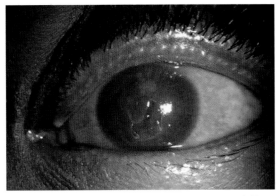

Fig. 3.4 Corneal shield ulcer in vernal keratoconjunctivitis.

Stevens–Johnson Syndrome (Erythema Multiforme Major)

Key Facts

- Acute inflammatory disease affecting skin and mucous membranes
- Mortality rate approaches 15%
- Secondary to certain drugs, vaccines, and infections
- Edematous or bullous skin lesions secondary to angiitis, causing concentric rings
- Prodrome of chills with pharyngitis, tachypnea, and tachycardia
- Bullous lesions then develop, followed by rupture, ulceration, then membrane formation

Clinical Findings

- Edema, erythema, and crusting of eyelids
- Vesicles or bullae of palpebral conjunctiva
- Watery mucoid discharge with membranes or pseudomembranes
- Symblepharon formation may occur
- **Late complications include:**
  - ectropion • entropion • symblepharon • trichiasis
- Severe dry eye secondary to conjunctival goblet cell destruction

Ancillary Testing

- Conjunctival biopsy

Differential Diagnosis

- Allergic conjunctivitis
- Kawasaki syndrome

Treatment

- Treat underlying cause (e.g. antivirals if herpes virus infection)
- Systemic corticosteroids controversial
- Early intervention important to prevent late complications
- Ocular lubricants
- Glass rod to lyse symblepharon formations
- Symblepharon ring
- Limbal transplantation and/or amniotic membrane grafting
- Treat any concomitant bacterial secondary infection

Prognosis

- Depends on extent of symblepharon formation and late complications, including dry eye and entropion or ectropion formation

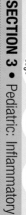

SECTION 3 • Pediatric: Inflammatory

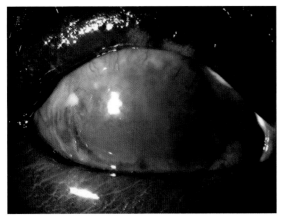

Fig. 3.5 Skin and lid lesions in acute Stevens–Johnson syndrome.

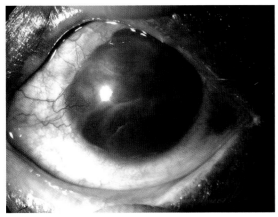

Fig. 3.6 Keratitis with conjunctival inflammation and necrosis in acute Stevens–Johnson syndrome. (From Taylor D, Hoyt CS 2005 Pediatric Ophthalmology and Strabismus, 3rd edn. Saunders, London.)

Kawasaki Syndrome

Key Facts

- Mucocutaneous lymph node syndrome
- Cause unknown
- Age <5 years in 85% of patients
- **Febrile illness lasting >5 days in association with:**
  - bilateral conjunctivitis
  - strawberry tongue, injected or fissured lips, or injected pharynx
  - rash
  - cervical lymphadenopathy
  - hand or foot edema, erythema of palms or soles, generalized or periungual desquamation
  - coronary artery aneurysm or coronary arteritis

Clinical Findings

- Self-limited anterior uveitis during acute phase
- Conjunctival scarring rare
- Retinal ischemia

Ancillary Testing

- Echocardiography

Differential Diagnosis

- Allergic conjunctivitis
- Stevens–Johnson syndrome

Treatment

- Aspirin
- Intravenous gamma globulin to shorten acute phase and prevent some coronary damage
- Topical corticosteroid and cycloplegic for anterior uveitis
- Supportive
- Systemic corticosteroids contraindicated because of increased risk of coronary artery aneurysm

Prognosis

- Depends on extent of systemic complications, with 1–2% risk of sudden death from coronary disease

Anterior Uveitis Secondary to Juvenile Rheumatoid Arthritis

Key Facts

- Uveitis associated with juvenile rheumatoid arthritis (JRA) • In children, antinuclear antibody (ANA)–positive, rheumatoid factor (RF)–negative • Usually diagnosed within 7 years of onset of arthritis • Uveitis uncommon before onset of arthritis • More common in females • Ocular symptoms of blurred vision and photophobia may not be present • Typically pauciarticular arthritis in children

Clinical Findings

- Anterior segment inflammatory cells and flare seen on slit-lamp examination • Band keratopathy, anterior segment synechiae, heterochromia iridis, and cystoid macular edema may be present • Reduction of visual acuity depends on extent of disease • Hypotony

Ancillary Testing

- ANA • RF

Differential Diagnosis

- **Uveitis associated with:**
  - trauma • sarcoid • Lyme disease • other spondyloarthropathies

Treatment

- Topical corticosteroids • Topical short-acting cycloplegic agents to prevent synechiae formation • Systemic corticosteroids or immunosuppressants (methotrexate or cyclosporine)

Prognosis

- Depends on extent of corneal and anterior segment disease at presentation • Aggressive topical and systemic treatment important to eliminate or significantly reduce anterior segment inflammation • Long-term complications of corticosteroids to eye include glaucoma and cataract formation

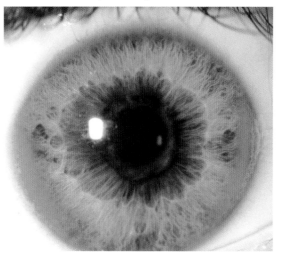

Fig. 3.7 Pupillary membrane extending from the iris margin in JRA uveitis. (From Taylor D, Hoyt CS 2005 Pediatric Ophthalmology and Strabismus, 3rd edn. Saunders, London.)

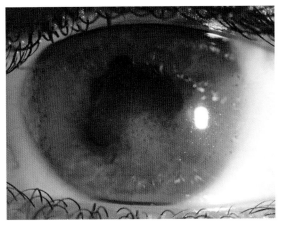

Fig. 3.8 Mild band keratopathy and posterior synechiae in JRA uveitis. (From Taylor D, Hoyt CS 2005 Pediatric Ophthalmology and Strabismus, 3rd edn. Saunders, London.)

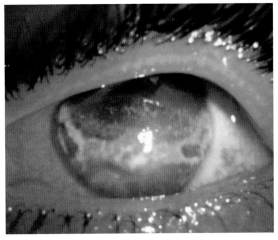

Fig. 3.9 Severe band keratopathy in juvenile rheumatoid arthritis uveitis. (From Taylor D, Hoyt CS 2005 Pediatric Ophthalmology and Strabismus, 3rd edn. Saunders, London.)

Pars Planitis (Intermediate Uveitis)

Key Facts

- Gradual onset of inflammation in region of peripheral retina and pars plana
- 25% of uveitis in pediatric age group
- **Composed of:**
  - mononuclear cells • occasional fibroblasts • hyperplastic non-pigmented ciliary epithelial cells
- Venous sheathing with lymphocytes
- In severe cases, fibroglial proliferation at vitreous base with neovascularization

Clinical Findings

- White opacities (snow banks) in region of peripheral retina and pars plana
- 75% bilateral
- Initial peripheral perivasculitis with exudate inferiorly that then extends nasally, temporally, and posteriorly
- **Development of:**
  - cystoid macular edema • papillitis • posterior subcapsular cataract
- Glaucoma and exudative retinal detachment may occur

Ancillary Testing

- Angiotensin-converting enzyme level and chest x-ray to rule out sarcoiditis

Differential Diagnosis

- Infectious chorioretinitis
- Retinitis pigmentosa
- Coats disease
- Retinopathy of prematurity
- Late onset retinoblastoma

Treatment

- Topical or periocular injections of corticosteroid
- Systemic corticosteroids or other immunosuppressants, including methotrexate or cyclosporine
- Transscleral diathermy and cryotherapy
- May require pars plana vitrectomy

Prognosis

- Depends on timely vigorous treatment or development of complications
- 10% self-limited course
- 60% prolonged course without exacerbations
- 30% chronic, smoldering course with exacerbations

SECTION 3 • Pediatric: Inflammatory

Orbital Pseudotumor

Key Facts
- Also known as idiopathic orbital inflammatory disease
- **Acute ocular pain associated with:**
  - headache • fever • nausea and vomiting • lethargy • possible diplopia
- More common in females
- Can be bilateral and episodic

Clinical Findings
- Proptosis
- Lid and conjunctival swelling and injection
- Possible motility disturbance
- Uveitis may be present

Ancillary Testing
- Full ophthalmic examination including visual acuity and extraocular motility evaluation
- Hertel exophthalmometry to measure extent of proptosis
- CT or MRI scan showing increased orbital fat density, thickening of extraocular muscle and tendons

Differential Diagnosis
- Orbital cellulitis
- Orbital mass
- Thyroid orbitopathy
- Orbital congestion secondary to cavernous sinus lesion

Treatment
- Orbital biopsy may be needed to establish or confirm diagnosis
- Systemic corticosteroid or immunosuppressants

Prognosis
- Depends on response of inflammation to medical treatment

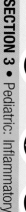

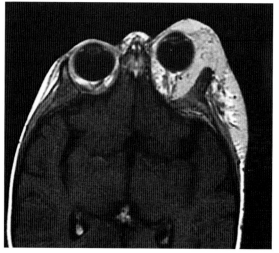

Fig. 3.10 Axial T₁ MRI with gadolinium contrast, showing enhancement of orbital pseudotumor.

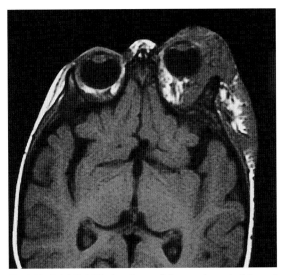

Fig. 3.11 Axial T₁ MRI showing soft tissue characteristics of orbital pseudotumor.

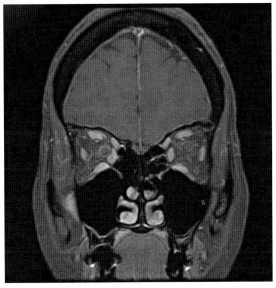

Fig. 3.12 Coronal T₁ fat saturation MRI with gadolinium, showing right medial and inferior rectus thickening along with optic nerve sheath enhancement in orbital myositis.

Section 4

Pediatric: Congenital Anomalies

Axenfeld–Rieger Syndrome

Key Facts

- Anterior segment dysgenesis with peripheral developmental abnormality
- Associated with glaucoma
- **Previously separated into:**
  - Axenfeld anomaly • Rieger anomaly • Rieger syndrome

Clinical Findings

- Microcornea or megalocornea
- Anterior displaced Schwalbe's line (posterior embryotoxin) with attached iris strands
- Smooth, cryptless iris surface with high iris insertion
- Iris hypoplasia ranges from mild stromal thinning to hole formation, corectopia, and ectropion uveae
- 50% associated glaucoma
- Facial bone and teeth defects
- Hypospadias, redundant periumbilical skin

Ancillary Testing

- Corneal pachymetry, visual field, and optical coherence tomography testing if glaucoma
- Genetic testing for RIEG1/PITX2 and FKHL7 mutations
- Evaluate family members—primarily autosomal dominant

Differential Diagnosis

- Aniridia
- Juvenile or congenital glaucoma
- Albinism
- Microphthalmia
- Isolated megalocornea or microcornea
- Peters anomaly

Treatment

- Fully correct refractive error
- Treat underlying amblyopia
- Monitor for glaucoma

Prognosis

- **Depends on:**
  - degree of abnormalities • compliance with treatment of glaucoma, if present

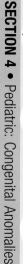

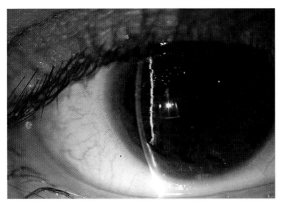

Fig. 4.1 Anterior displaced Schwalbe's line (posterior embryotoxin) with attached iris strand in Axenfeld–Rieger syndrome.

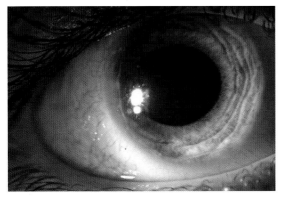

Fig. 4.2 Iris corectopia in Axenfeld–Rieger syndrome.

Peters Anomaly

Key Facts

- Anterior segment dysgenesis with central developmental abnormality leading to stromal opacification (leukoma)
- Local absence of Descemet's membrane
- **Syndrome includes:**
  - microphthalmia • linear skin lesions • cardiac arrhythmias

Clinical Findings

- Posterior corneal defect with stromal opacification (leukoma)
- Iris strands inserting into corneal defect
- Leukoma may become vascularized
- Adhesions of lens to corneal defect may also occur
- Glaucoma in 50% of cases
- May have anterior polar cataract
- Vision depends on location of corneal opacity (central versus paracentral)

Ancillary Testing

- Genetic and systemic work-up, especially if bilateral

Differential Diagnosis

- Central posterior keratoconus
- Sclerocornea
- Mucopolysaccharidosis and mucolipidosis
- Forceps injury
- Congenital hereditary endothelial dystrophy
- Corneal dermoid
- Congenital hereditary stromal dystrophy
- Infantile glaucoma
- Congenital rubella
- Microphthalmia

Treatment

- Fully correct refractive error
- Treat underlying amblyopia and glaucoma
- Lysis of adherent iris strands may improve corneal opacity
- Consider corneal transplant if bilateral central opacities affecting vision
  - Transplantation for unilateral opacity is controversial given the high incidence of graft failure and severity of induced amblyopia
  - Postoperative care requires frequent follow-up

Prognosis

- **Depends on:**
  - density and location of corneal opacity (central versus paracentral)
  - response to glaucoma treatments
- Stromal opacity may decrease over time

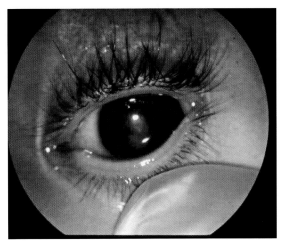

Fig. 4.3 Central leukoma Peters anomaly.

Mucopolysaccharidosis and Mucolipidosis

Key Facts

- Deficiency of enzymes catalyzing stepwise degradation of mucopolysaccharides (glycosaminoglycans) • Accumulation of glycosaminoglycans in ocular structures • Six types, all autosomal recessive except mucopolysaccharidosis (MPS) type 2 (X-linked recessive)
- **MPS type IH:**
  - deficiency of α-L-iduronidase
  - onset between 6 months and 2 years
  - patients rarely live past age 10
  - coarse facial features, enlarged tongue, hepatosplenomegaly, cardiac disease, developmental delay, dysostosis multiplex
- **MPS type IS:**
  - similar to MPS type IH except normal stature and intelligence
- **MPS type II (Hunter):**
  - deficiency of iduronate sulfatase
- **MPS type III (Sanfilippo):**
  - deficiency of heparin N-sulfatase or N-acetyl-α-D-glucosaminidase
- **MPS type IV (Morquio):**
  - deficiency of N-acetyl-gluctosamine-6-sulfatase or β-galactosidase
  - inability to degrade keratin sulfate
  - dwarfism, skeletal abnormalities, normal intelligence
- **MPS type VI (Maroteaux–Lamy):**
  - deficiency of arylsulfatase B
  - inability to degrade dermatan sulfate
  - similar to MPS type II except normal intelligence
- **MPS type VII (Sly):**
  - deficiency of β-glucuronidase

Clinical Findings

- Corneal clouding in all types except MPS type II • Papilledema and glaucoma in MPS types I and VI • Optic atrophy in MPS types I, II, and VI • Retinal pigmentary degeneration in MPS types I–III

Ancillary Testing

- Full systemic work-up • Genetic evaluation

Differential Diagnosis

- Central posterior keratoconus • Sclerocornea • Congenital hereditary endothelial dystrophy • Forceps injury • Peters anomaly • Corneal dermoid • Congenital hereditary stromal dystrophy • Infantile glaucoma • Congenital rubella

Treatment

- Corneal transplantation • Glaucoma treatment • Treatment of systemic disorder with possible enzyme replacement, stem cell transplantation, or allogenic bone marrow transplantation, dependent on type

Prognosis

- Depends on type and possible systemic treatments

Table 4.1 MPS disorders and underlying enzyme deficiencies

Type	Eponym	Stored material	Enzyme deficiency
MPS IH	Hurler	DS, HS	Iduronidase
MPS IS	Sheie	DS, HS	Iduronidase
MPS IH/S	Hurler-Sheie	DS, HS	Iduronidase
MPS II	Hunter (X-LR)	DS, HS	Iduronidase sulfate sulfatase
MPS IIIA	Sanfilipo	HS	Heparin N-sulfatase
MPS IIIB		HS	N-acetylglucosaminidase
MPS IIIC		HS	Acetyl-coenzyme-A-glucosaminidase-acetyltransferase
MPS IIID		HS	N-acetylglucosaminidase 6-sulfatase
MPS IVA	Morquio	–	Galactosamine-6-sulfatase
MPS IVB		–	β-galactosidase
MPS VI	Maroteaux-Lamy	DS	N-acetylglucosaminidase 4-sulfatase
MPS VIII	Sly	HS, CS, DS	β-glucuronidase

Table 4.1 (From Taylor D, Hoyt CS 2005 Pediatric Ophthalmology and Strabismus, 3rd edn. Saunders, London.)

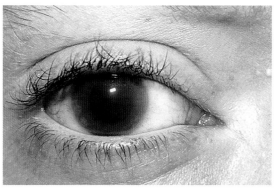

Fig. 4.4 Corneal clouding in MPS type IS. (From Taylor D, Hoyt CS 2005 Pediatric Ophthalmology and Strabismus, 3rd edn. Saunders, London.)

Congenital Hereditary Endothelial Dystrophy

Key Facts

- Diffuse corneal edema secondary to defect of corneal endothelium and Descemet's membrane
- Autosomal dominant and autosomal recessive, both on chromosome 20 but on different loci
- **Symptoms include:**
  - pain • tearing • photophobia

Clinical Findings

- Uniformly edematous cornea involving both epithelium and stroma
- Increased corneal thickness
- Nystagmus
- Usually presents at birth

Ancillary Testing

- Genetic work-up

Differential Diagnosis

- Central posterior keratoconus
- Sclerocornea
- Mucopolysaccharidosis and mucolipidosis
- Forceps injury
- Peters anomaly
- Corneal dermoid
- Congenital hereditary stromal dystrophy
- Infantile glaucoma
- Congenital rubella

Treatment

- Penetrating corneal transplantation successful in 60% of patients
- May be a role for endothelial keratoplasty in the future

Prognosis

- Depends on success and complication rate of corneal transplantation

SECTION 4 • Pediatric: Congenital Anomalies

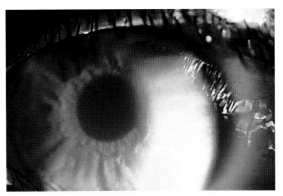

Fig. 4.5 Opaque cornea in congenital hereditary endothelial dystrophy (CHED). (From Taylor D, Hoyt CS 2005 Pediatric Ophthalmology and Strabismus, 3rd edn. Saunders, London.)

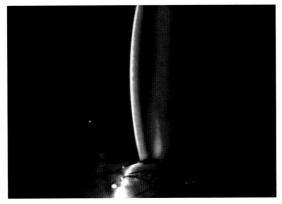

Fig. 4.6 Opaque and thickened cornea on slit-lamp illumination in CHED. (From Taylor D, Hoyt CS 2005 Pediatric Ophthalmology and Strabismus, 3rd edn. Saunders, London.)

Limbal Dermoid

Key Facts

- Choristoma composed of keratinized epithelium overlying fibrofatty tissue
- **May contain:**
  - hair follicles • sebaceous glands • sweat glands
- May enlarge slowly during puberty or after trauma
- May cause corneal astigmatism and anisometropic amblyopia

Clinical Findings

- Typically 5–10 mm in diameter, involving inferotemporal limbus
- Extends into corneal stroma and sclera but rarely full thickness
- Lipoid infiltration extending into corneal stroma at leading edge
- **Goldenhar syndrome (oculoauriculovertebral dysplasia):**
  - epibulbar dermoid, preauricular appendages, vertebral anomalies
  - 25% bilateral
  - 25% upper eyelid coloboma
  - associated with colobomas of upper eyelid, iris, and choroid
  - micrognathia, facial asymmetry, and dental abnormalities

Ancillary Testing

- Genetic and full systemic work-up

Differential Diagnosis

- Conjunctival epithelial cyst
- Conjunctival nevi
- Pterygium

Treatment

- Excision of large symptomatic lesions
  - May extend full thickness and require corneoscleral patch graft
- Correct ansiometropia and amblyopia with glasses and patching

Prognosis

- Depends on size of lesion and consequent visual disturbance
- Excision complications include corneal perforation and persistent corneal scarring and may not improve underlying astigmatism

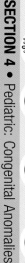

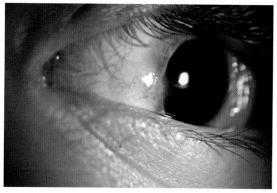

Fig. 4.7 Limbal dermoid.

Congenital Glaucoma (Primary Congenital Glaucoma)

Key Facts

- Structural or intrinsic abnormality of aqueous outflow
- 1 : 10 000 births
- Most bilateral
- 10% familial, usually autosomal recessive with variable penetrance (GLC3 gene, chromosome 2p21)
- Autosomal dominant chromosome 1p36
- Possible developmental arrest of anterior chamber tissue derived from neural crest tissue
- **Presenting signs:**
  - epiphora • photophobia • blepharospasm

Clinical Findings

- Progressive corneal edema with breaks in Descemet's membrane (Haab striae)
- Elevated IOP, typically non-sedated between 30 and 40 mmHg
- Corneal enlargement
- **Gonioscopy:**
  - normal landmarks difficult to recognize with decreased transparency of tissues over scleral spur and ciliary body band
- Diminished width of trabecular meshwork and ciliary body
- Abnormal increased cup : disc ratio (>0.3 typically), which may improve with lowering IOP
- Buphthalmos, scleral thinning with myopia, and spontaneous lens dislocation can occur without treatment

Ancillary Testing

- **Full ophthalmic examination, usually under anesthesia, including:**
  - measurement of corneal diameter
  - IOP with gonioscopy and fundoscopy
- Note that all anesthetics lower IOP except ketamine, chloral hydrate, and nitrous oxide
  - Sevoflurane and other inhalational agents may substantially lower IOP

Differential Diagnosis

- **Primary developmental glaucoma:**
  - Sturge–Weber syndrome • neurofibromatosis • aniridia • Peters anomaly • sclerocornea • posterior polymorphous dystrophy • congenital hereditary endothelial dystrophy • congenital rubella • Lowe (oculocerebrorenal) syndrome
- **Secondary glaucoma:**
  - angle recession post trauma • uveitis or secondary to intraocular inflammation • secondary to intraocular neoplasm • steroid-induced • aphakia

Treatment

- **Medical (rarely successful in long term):**
  - carbonic anhydrase inhibitors (oral acetazolamide 10–20 mg/kg per day in divided doses, dorzolamide hydrochloride ophthalmic solution 2.0% t.i.d., or brinzolamide ophthalmic solution)
  - topical beta blockers (timolol maleate or betaxolol)

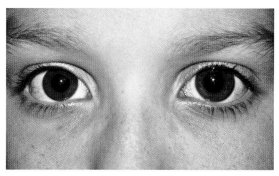

Fig. 4.8 Left buphthalmos in congenital glaucoma. (From Taylor D, Hoyt CS 2005 Pediatric Ophthalmology and Strabismus, 3rd edn. Saunders, London.)

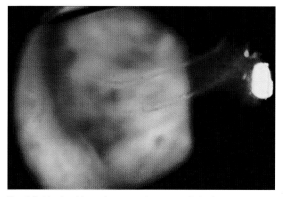

Fig. 4.9 Haab striae of cornea in congenital glaucoma. (From Taylor D, Hoyt CS 2005 Pediatric Ophthalmology and Strabismus, 3rd edn. Saunders, London.)

- • miotics or adrenergic agents less effective (central nervous system depression with brimonidine tartrate)
  - • prostaglandin (latanoprost shows variable response)
- **Surgical (treatment of choice):**
  - • goniotomy
  - • trabeculotomy
  - • trabeculectomy
  - • Seton implant (Molteno, Baerveldt, Ahmed)
  - • cycloablation (Nd : YAG, diode laser, cyclocryotherapy, endoscopy)
- Simultaneous treatment of myopia and amblyopia

Prognosis

- In 80% of cases presenting from 3 months to 1 year old, IOP controlled with one or two surgical procedures
- Trabeculotomy with mitomycin-C successful in 50–90% of cases, but high long-term risk of bleb leaks and endophthalmitis
- Success rate of Seton implant is 60–85%
- 33% success rate for cycloablation, with retreatments commonly required
- 10% complication of phthisis
- Trans-scleral laser cycloablation and endoscopy success about 50%, with 70% retreatment rate in former
- Prognosis poor if glaucoma presents at birth, with half the eyes becoming blind

Aniridia

Key Facts

- Absent or rudimentary iris is hallmark, but iris anatomy can be quite variable
- Bilateral, with gene defect on chromosome 11
- Autosomal dominant but can be sporadic
- Two-thirds of children have affected parents
- Poor visual acuity with nystagmus and photophobia common

Clinical Findings

- Iris anatomy ranges from absent or rudimentary stump to phenotypically normal
- Persistent pupillary membranes
- Corneal pannus that progresses centrally throughout patient's life (aniridic keratopathy)
- Anterior polar cataracts
- Foveal and optic nerve hypoplasia and nystagmus
- Wilms, aniridia, genitourinary malformations, and mental retardation (WAGR) complex

Ancillary Testing

- Chromosome analysis
- Oncology evaluation and abdominal ultrasound if Wilms tumor gene present

Differential Diagnosis

- Albinism
- Congenital glaucoma or cataracts
- Congenital nystagmus
- Optic nerve hypoplasia

Treatment

- Fully correct refractive error in both eyes with glasses and treat underlying amblyopia
- Monitor for development of elevated IOP and glaucoma
- Corneal pannus formation progressive and may improve after limbal stem cell tranplantation
- Sunglasses

Prognosis

- **Depends on:**
  - degree of nystagmus • foveal hypoplasia • development of glaucoma, cataract, and aniridic keratopathy

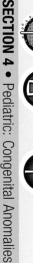

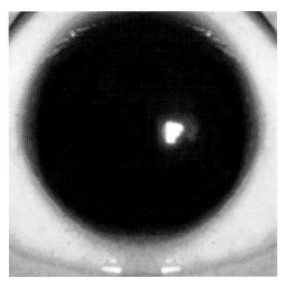

Fig. 4.10 Absent iris in aniridia.

Albinism

Key Facts

- Congenital reduction or absence of intracellular melanin pigment • **Ocular albinism:** localized to eye • Oculocutaneous albinism (OCA) involves eye, skin, and hair • Abnormal visual pathways with excess number of neurons crossing in chiasm • **OCA type 1:** reduced or absent tyrosinase activity • **OCA type 2:** P gene defect, tyrosinase-positive • **OCA type 3:** all autosomal recessive • Oculocutaneous and X-linked ocular are most common
- **Chediak–Higashi syndrome:**
  - neutropenia with recurrent infection, thrombocytopenia, anemia • leukemia, lymphoma
- **Hermansky–Pudlak syndrome:**
  - high frequency in Puerto Rico • platelet bleeding disorder

Clinical Findings

- Acuity from 20/40 to 20/200 • Nystagmus • Iris transillumination defects • Retinal pigment deficiency • Foveal hypoplasia or aplasia • High refractive error • Frequent strabismus

Ancillary Testing

- Genetic testing with chromosome analysis • White blood cell and platelet count • Bleeding time

Differential Diagnosis

- Congenital nystagmus • Retinal disorders such as gyrate atrophy and cone rod dystrophy • Congenital glaucoma or cataracts • Optic nerve hypoplasia • Gyrate atrophy • Aniridia

Treatment

- Skin and eye protection from sun exposure • Fully correct refractive error in both eyes with glasses and treat underlying amblyopia

Prognosis

- **Depends on:**
  - degree of nystagmus • extent of foveal and optic nerve hypoplasia

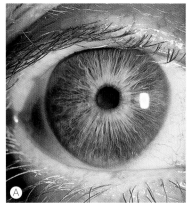
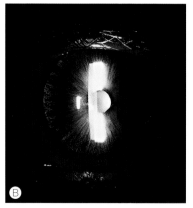

Fig. 4.11 Moderate transillumination on retroillumination in a blue-eyed albino carrier. (From Taylor D, Hoyt CS 2005 Pediatric Ophthalmology and Strabismus, 3rd edn. Saunders, London.)

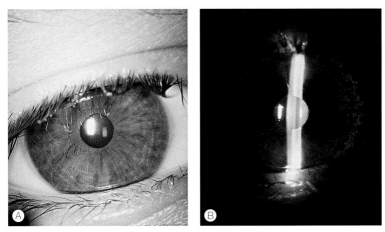

Fig. 4.12 (**A**) Brown iris in X-linked ocular albinism with reduced vision and nystagmus. (**B**) Marked iris transillumination in the same patient. (From Taylor D, Hoyt CS 2005 Pediatric Ophthalmology and Strabismus, 3rd edn. Saunders, London.)

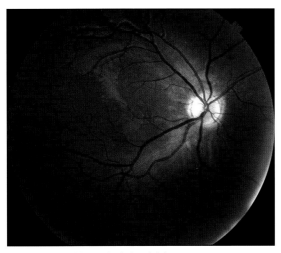

Fig. 4.13 Foveal hypoplasia in albinism.

Iris Coloboma

Key Facts

- Defect in closure of embryonic fissure during fifth week of gestation
- Association with retinal and optic nerve coloboma, leading to reduced acuity and, if bilateral, nystagmus
- Associated microphthalmia, autosomal dominant in 20% of cases
- Association with ocular coloboma, heart defects, choanal atresia, mental retardation, and genitourinary and ear anomalies (CHARGE)
- **Association with:**
  - trisomy 13 or 18 • Wolf–Hirschhorn syndrome • 11q-, 13r, Turner, and Klinefelter syndrome
- **If additional uveal coloboma, consider the following syndromes:**
  - Aicardi • Warburg • Rubinstein–Taybi • linear sebaceous nevus • Goldenhar

Clinical Findings

- Typical inferonasal keyhole-shaped defect
- Lens zonules may also be affected, leading to flattening of lens without dislocation
- Possible retinal and optic nerve coloboma

Ancillary Testing

- Chromosome analysis, especially if other organ system involvement

Differential Diagnosis

- Ectopia lentis et pupillae
- Iridocorneal endothelium syndrome
- Traumatic iris tear
- Aniridia

Treatment

- Fully correct refractive error in both eyes with glasses if lenticular astigmatism

Prognosis

- Excellent visual prognosis if isolated iris coloboma
- Visual potential depends on extent of retinal, optic nerve, and other organ system involvement

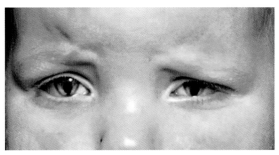

Fig. 4.14 Bilateral iris colobomas. (From Spalton D et al. 2005 Atlas of Clinical Ophthalmology, 3rd edn. Mosby, London.)

Juvenile Xanthogranuloma

Key Facts

- Non-neoplastic histiocytic proliferation
- Orange or tan small round papules on skin
- Occurs in infants younger that 2 years
- Spontaneous hyphema
- Secondary glaucoma with pain and photophobia

Clinical Findings

- Localized yellow or brown iris mass
- Iris heterochromia secondary to diffuse mass
- Spontaneous hyphema
- Elevated IOP

Ancillary Testing

- Pathology of lesion shows Touton giant cells
- Complete dermatologic examination

Differential Diagnosis

- Autoimmune associated uveitis
- Traumatic iritis
- Uveal melanoma
- Iris nevi
- Lisch's nodules
- Medulloepithelioma

Treatment

- Topical corticosteroids
- Glaucoma treatment
- Surgical excision of lesion or radiation if intractable glaucoma

Prognosis

- Self-limited because lesion typically regresses by age 5
- If hyphema obscures visual axis for extended period, amblyopia could be present once hyphema resorbs

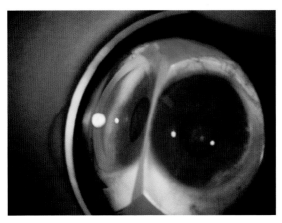

Fig. 4.15 Gonioscopy view in juvenile xanthogranuloma, showing the angle filled with yellowish xanthogranuloma material. (From Taylor D, Hoyt CS 2005 Pediatric Ophthalmology and Strabismus, 3rd edn. Saunders, London.)

Persistent Pupillary Membrane

Key Facts

- Common developmental abnormality of iris
- Rarely causes visual abnormality
- May adhere to anterior lens capsule, leading to cataract

Clinical Findings

- Papillary remnant strands exiting from iris across pupil
- Rare anterior polar cataract

Ancillary Testing

- Gonioscopy

Differential Diagnosis

- Axenfeld–Rieger syndrome
- Peters anomaly
- Posterior synechiae secondary to iridocyclitis
- Iridocorneal endothelium syndrome

Treatment

- Correct refractive error
- Cataract extraction if visually significant

Prognosis

- Excellent
- Rarely of visual significance

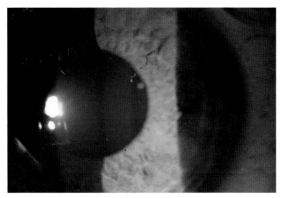

Fig. 4.16 Persistent papillary membrane extending from mid iris into anterior chamber.

Spherophakia

Key Facts
- Congenital lens abnormality
- Lens may dislocate, causing glaucoma

Clinical Findings
- Lens that is more spherical and smaller than normal
- Lens may be dislocated with increased IOP
- Lenticular refractive error

Ancillary Testing
- Family history

Differential Diagnosis
- **Lens dislocation secondary to:**
  - Marfan syndrome • Weil–Marchesani syndrome • homocystinuria • syphilis • Ehlers–Danlos syndrome • aniridia • coloboma • trauma • hereditary ectopia lentis

Treatment
- Correct refractive error
- Lensectomy if lens dislocated or uncorrectable refractive error

Prognosis
- Excellent if refractive error correctable
- Depends on extent of glaucomatous damage if lens dislocated

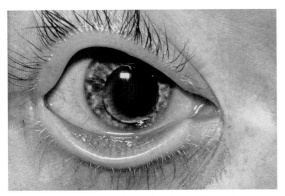
Fig. 4.17 Microspherophakia with anterior dislocation.
(From Taylor D, Hoyt CS 2005 Pediatric Ophthalmology
and Strabismus, 3rd edn. Saunders, London.)

Marfan Syndrome

Key Facts

- Abnormality of fibrillin structure
- **Involves ocular, musculoskeletal, and cardiovascular systems:**
  - tall, with long limbs • arachnodactyly • loose joints • chest deformity (pectus excavatum) • aortic root enlargement • aortic aneurysm formation • floppy mitral valve

Clinical Findings

- Progressive upward dislocation of lens
- Visible intact lens zonules
- **Myopia:**
  - increased axial length
- Increased risk of retinal detachment

Ancillary Testing

- Family history
- A-scan ultrasound
- Cardiology evaluation to include cardiac echo and electrocardiogram

Differential Diagnosis

- Lens dislocation secondary to spherophakia
- Weil–Marchesani syndrome
- homocystinuria
- syphilis
- Ehlers–Danlos syndrome
- aniridia
- coloboma
- trauma
- hereditary ectopia lentis

Treatment

- Correct refractive error
- Lensectomy if lens dislocated or uncorrectable refractive error
- Treat amblyopia
- Monitor for retinal detachment
- Safety glasses during sports to prevent further lens dislocation from accidental eye trauma

Prognosis

- Life expectancy reduced secondary to cardiovascular abnormalities
- **Visual prognosis depends on:**
  - early correction of refractive error • treatment of amblyopia • retinal detachment, if occurs

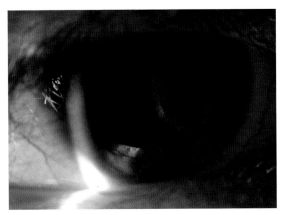

Fig. 4.18 Lens dislocation in the right eye in Marfan syndrome.

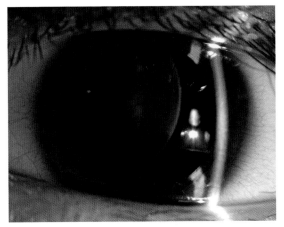

Fig. 4.19 Lens dislocation in the left eye in Marfan syndrome.

Persistent Hyperplastic Primary Vitreous

Key Facts

- Typically unilateral congenital abnormality of incomplete regression of fetal vasculature
- Most commonly associated with cataract and microphthalmia
- Also called persistent fetal vasculature

Clinical Findings

- Cataract with present vascular remnants
- Microphthalmia
- Retrolental fibrovascular membrane
- Vascular stalk can extend from posterior lens capsule to optic disc
- Retina and optic nerve abnormality, including traction or dysplasia
- Bergmeister papillae (stalk remnant confined to optic disc)
- Mittendorf dot (small remnant confined to lens capsule)
- Anisometropia and strabismus common

Ancillary Testing

- Complete ophthalmic examination including retinoscopy
- If unable to view posterior pole or perform retinoscopy because of cataract, then A and B scan would determine axial length and may show optic nerve or retinal dysplasia

Differential Diagnosis

- Microphthalmia
- Congenital cataract
- Stage 4 retinopathy of prematurity
- Anisometropic pathologic myopia

Treatment

- Fully correct refractive error in both eyes with glasses
  - Protective lens if no refractive error or visual potential
- Treat amblyopia
- Consider cataract extraction with or without vitrectomy depending on extent of posterior involvement

Prognosis

- **Depends on:**
  - degree of abnormalities • compliance with treatment

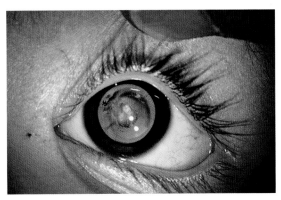

Fig. 4.20 Small persistent fetal vascular with cataract.
(From Taylor D, Hoyt CS 2005 Pediatric Ophthalmology
and Strabismus, 3rd edn. Saunders, London.)

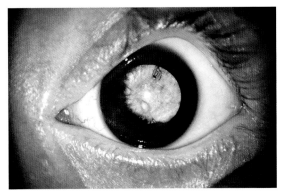

Fig. 4.21 Marked persistant fetal vasculature with multiple
vessels between a large fibrous plaque, lens, and the iris.
(From Taylor D, Hoyt CS 2005 Pediatric Ophthalmology
and Strabismus, 3rd edn. Saunders, London.)

Retinopathy of Prematurity

Key Facts

- Proliferative retinal vascular disorder affecting markedly premature infants
- **Risk of retinopathy of prematurity (ROP):**
  - birth weight 1250 g (47%)
  - birth weight 750 g (90%)
- Usually becomes apparent 32–34 weeks post conception regardless of gestational age

Clinical Findings

- International classification
  Zone (anterior posterior location)
  - 1: circle within posterior pole with radius twice the nerve–macula distance
  - 2: edge of zone 1 to a circle with radius equal to distance from optic nerve to nasal ora serrata
  - 3: residual crescent anterior to zone 2
  Clock hours (circumferential extent)
  Stage (severity)
  - 1: demarcation line
  - 2: ridge
  - 3: ridge with extraretinal fibrovascular proliferation
  - 4: subtotal retinal detachment (A, extrafoveal; B, including fovea)
  - 5: total funnel retinal detachment
  Plus disease (presence of vascular dilation and tortuosity in posterior pole)
- **Regressed ROP:**
  - myopia • vitreous membranes • equatorial retinal folds at past demarcation line • retinal dragging • lattice-like degeneration with retinal breaks
- **Unfavorable outcome after treatment:**
  - macular fold • progression of disease • cataract • microphthalmia • glaucoma • phthisis

Ancillary Testing

- Low vision evaluation
- B-scan ultrasound if unable to view retina

Differential Diagnosis

- Familial exudative vitreoretinopathy
- Coats disease
- Retinoblastoma
- Incontinentia pigmenti
- Toxoplasmosis or *Toxocara*
- Norrie disease

Treatment

- **Cryotherapy for Retinopathy of Prematurity (Cryo-ROP) study:**
  - treat threshold disease with five contiguous or eight cumulative clock hours for stage 3 ROP, zone 1 or 2 disease with plus
- **Indirect laser photocoagulation:**
  - similar results to Cryo-ROP

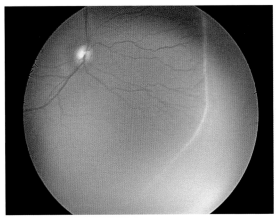

Fig. 4.22 ROP stages 1 and 2. Stage 1 (demarcation line) is in the lower part, but the line becomes thicker (ridge) toward the top of the image. (From Taylor D, Hoyt CS 2005 Pediatric Ophthalmology and Strabismus, 3rd edn. Saunders, London.)

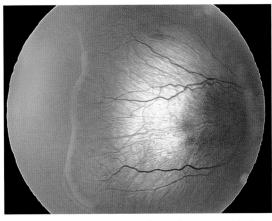

Fig. 4.23 ROP stages 2 and 3. Stage 2 at top and bottom of the image, with about one clock hour of mild stage 3 disease that curls away from the ridge at its lower edge. (From Taylor D, Hoyt CS 2005 Pediatric Ophthalmology and Strabismus, 3rd edn. Saunders, London.)

- **Early Treatment for Retinopathy of Prematurity (ET-ROP) study:**
  - treatment of high-risk prethreshold
  - zone 1, any stage with plus disease
  - zone 1, stage 3 ROP with or without plus disease
  - zone 2, stage 2 or 3 ROP with plus disease
- Scleral buckle for stage 4 detachments and shallow, open funnel stage 5 detachments
- Vitrectomy with or without lensectomy for more extensive detachments
- Low vision aids

Prognosis
- **Cryo-ROP:**
  - for infants with threshold ROP, unfavorable outcome defined as vision less than 20/200 at age 3.5 years
  - 22% with cryotherapy treatment, 43% observed
  - despite anatomical surgical success for stage 4 and 5, development of useful vision is obtained in minority of patients
- **ET-ROP study:**
  - reduction of unfavorable visual outcomes to 14.5% and structural outcomes to 9.1% in treatment of high-risk prethreshold with laser

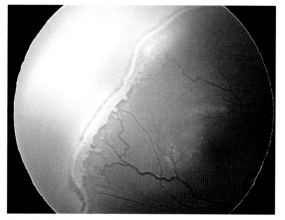

Fig. 4.24 ROP stage 3. Note the peripheral tortuosity and dilation as the vessels become close to the neovascular ridge. (From Taylor D, Hoyt CS 2005 Pediatric Ophthalmology and Strabismus, 3rd edn. Saunders, London.)

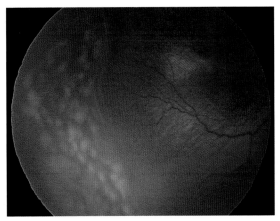

Fig. 4.25 Fresh laser lesions applied anterior to the neovascular ridge. (From Taylor D, Hoyt CS 2005 Pediatric Ophthalmology and Strabismus, 3rd edn. Saunders, London.)

Table 4.2 Stages of ROP

Stage 1	Demarcation line
Stage 2	Ridge
Stage 3	Ridge with extraretinal fibrovascular proliferation
Stage 4	Subtotal retinal detachment
	Extrafoveal
	Retinal detachment including fovea
Stage 5	Total retinal detachment

Funnel	
Anterior	**Posterior**
Open	Open
Narrow	Narrow
Open	Narrow
Narrow	Open

From Committee for Classification of Retinopathy of Prematurity

Table 4.2 (From Taylor D, Hoyt CS 2005 Pediatric Ophthalmology and Strabismus, 3rd edn. Saunders, London.)

Leber Congenital Amaurosis

Key Facts

- Congenital retinal disorder of rods and cones • Autosomal recessive • Eye poking; oculodigital reflex • Absence of photoreceptors histologically • Mutation of RETGC1, RPE65, and CRX genes
- **Associated with:**
  - polycystic kidney • osteopetrosis • cleft palate • seizures • hydrocephalus

Clinical Findings

- Nystagmus • Vision 20/200 to bare light perception • Hyperopia with sluggish pupils most common • Early normal-appearing retina
- **With time:**
  - development of retinal bone spicules • attenuation of arterioles • optic disc pallor
- Chorioretinal atrophy with white dots • Cataracts, keratoconus, keratoglobus

Ancillary Testing

- **Electroretinogram:**
  - extinguished at birth
- Low vision evaluation • Genetic and neurologic evaluation • Measurement of serum phytanic acid and evaluation for acanthocytes to rule out Refsum disease and abetalipoproteinemia

Differential Diagnosis

- **Refsum disease:**
  - infantile phytanic acid storage disease
- **Bassen–Kornzweig syndrome:**
  - abetalipoproteinemia
- **Batten disease:**
  - ceroid lipofuscinosis
- Achromatopsia • Blue cone monochromatism • Congenital stationary night blindness • Foveal hypoplasia • Aicardi syndrome

Treatment

- Correct refractive error if present • Low vision aids • No known treatment of retinal abnormality

Prognosis

- Poor visual acuity

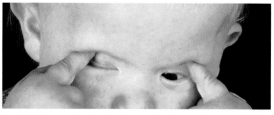

Fig. 4.26 Oculodigital sign (eye poking) in Leber congenital amaurosis. This can result in orbital fat atrophy and enophthalmos. (From Taylor D, Hoyt CS 2005 Pediatric Ophthalmology and Strabismus, 3rd edn. Saunders, London.)

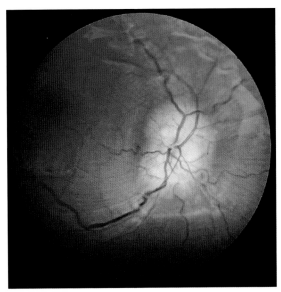

Fig. 4.27 High hypermetropia and pseudopapilledema in Leber congenital amaurosis (right eye). (From Taylor D, Hoyt CS 2005 Pediatric Ophthalmology and Strabismus, 3rd edn. Saunders, London.)

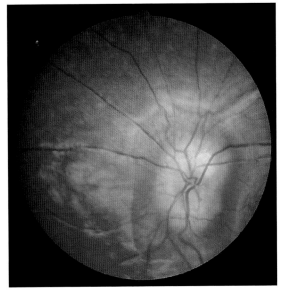

Fig. 4.28 High hypermetropia and pseudopapilledema in Leber congenital amaurosis (left eye). (From Taylor D, Hoyt CS 2005 Pediatric Ophthalmology and Strabismus, 3rd edn. Saunders, London.)

Morning Glory Disc

Key Facts

- Congenital anomaly of optic disc and surrounding retina
- Central glial tissue, funnel-shaped peripapillary excavation with radial retinal blood vessels, and a wide annulus of chorioretinal pigmentary disturbance that resembles morning glory flower
- Basal encephalocele

Clinical Findings

- Optic disc enlargement and funnel-shaped excavation with central core of white glial tissue
- Contractile properties so that disc can appear to open and close
- Variably pigmented annulus of peripapillary subretinal tissue
- Retinal vessels enter and exit from border of defect
- Vessels frequently sheathed and straightened
- Non-rhegmatogenous posterior retinal detachment in 30% of patients
- Strabismus

Ancillary Testing

- Brain MRI scan

Differential Diagnosis

- Optic disc coloboma
- Optic pit
- Megalopapilla
- Peripapillary staphyloma

Treatment

- Correct refractive error, strabismus, and amblyopia if present
- **Treat retinal detachment:**
  - peripapillary laser and vitrectomy with air–gas/fluid exchange

Prognosis

- **Visual acuity typically ranges from counting fingers to 20/200, with case reports of 20/20 vision, but depends on:**
  - extent of optic nerve and macular involvement • serous retinal detachment

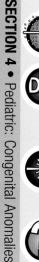

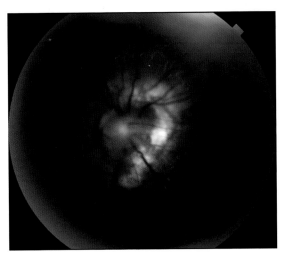

Fig. 4.29 Morning glory disc anomaly.

Optic Nerve Coloboma

Key Facts

- Defective embryogenesis in which fetal or choroidal fissure fails to close
- Eyelid coloboma may be isolated or associated with Goldenhar syndrome or craniofacial dysostosis
- Ocular coloboma with iris, lens, retina, or optic nerve involvement
- Association with coloboma, heart defects, choanal atresia, mental retardation, and genitourinary or ear anomalies (CHARGE)
- Unilateral or bilateral

Clinical Findings

- Eyelid notch
- Iris coloboma
- Segmental lens, retina, choroid, or optic nerve abnormality
- Microphthalmia
- Nystagmus if significant visual deprivation
- Astigmatism or myopia
- Leukocoria

Ancillary Testing

- Complete ophthalmic examination including retinoscopy
- B-scan ultrasound to evaluate for posterior cyst
- Genetic testing

Differential Diagnosis

- Anterior segment dysgenesis
- Retinopathy of prematurity, Coats disease, retinoblastoma
- Optic nerve pit or staphyloma

Treatment

- Fully correct refractive error in both eyes with glasses, protective lens if no visual potential
- Treat underlying amblyopia
- Scleral shell or orbital expander if microphthalmic
- Correct strabismus if present
- Monitor for retinal detachment

Prognosis

- **Depends on:**
  - degree of abnormalities • compliance with treatment

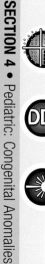

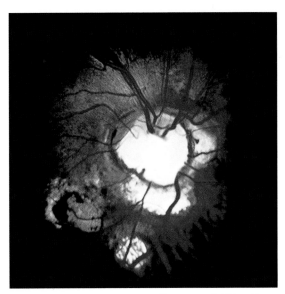

Fig. 4.30 Optic nerve coloboma. (Courtesy of William F. Hoyt, MD.)

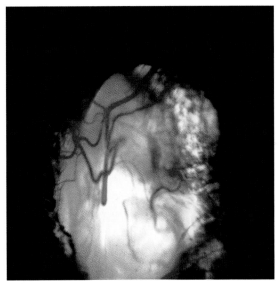

Fig. 4.31 Optic nerve and retinal coloboma. (Courtesy of William F. Hoyt, MD.)

Section 5

Pediatric: Hereditary Retinal Disorders

Sphingolipidoses

Key Facts

- Inherited disorder of sphingolipid degradation resulting in excessive intralysosomal accumulation
- Cherry red spot secondary to choroidal circulation view in fovea, where ganglion cells that accumulate sphingolipids are absent
- With death of ganglion cells, cherry red spot fades and optic atrophy develops along with nystagmus and retinal vessel attenuation
- G_{M2} type 1 gangliosidosis (Tay–Sachs disease):
  - hexosaminidase A deficiency
  - most common of the gangliosidoses occurring in persons of Ashkenazi Jewish descent
  - progressive neurodegeneration with spasticity and seizures
- G_{M2} type 2 gangliosidosis (Sandhoff disease):
  - hexosaminidase B deficiency
- G_{M1} type 1 gangliosidosis:
  - β-galactokinase deficiency
  - occasional corneal clouding and retinal hemorrhages
  - coarse facial features
  - hepatomegaly
- **Metochromatic leukodystrophy (arylsulfatase deficiency):**
  - demyelination from sulfatide accumulation and cerebellar atrophy
- **Niemann–Pick disease types A and B (sphingomyelinase deficiency):**
  - failure to thrive, with feeding difficulties
  - respiratory infections
  - hepatosplenomegaly
  - more prevalent in Ashkenazi Jewish population

Clinical Findings

- Rapid or slow neurodegeneration along with seizures, depending on type
- Cherry red spot
- Optic atrophy

Ancillary Testing

- Full systemic work-up
- Genetic evaluation

Differential Diagnosis

- **Other diseases with a cherry red spot:**
  - sialidosis types 1 and 2
  - mucolipidosis type 3
  - Farber disease

Treatment

- Limited treatments, mainly supportive
- Seizure control
- Possible bone marrow transplantation, depending on type

Prognosis

- Overall poor

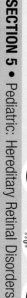

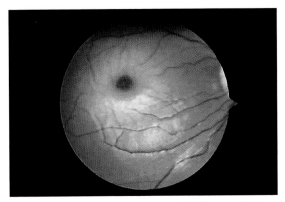

Fig. 5.1 Cherry red spot in a patient with Niemann–Pick disease. (From Taylor D, Hoyt CS 2005 Pediatric Ophthalmology and Strabismus, 3rd edn. Saunders, London.)

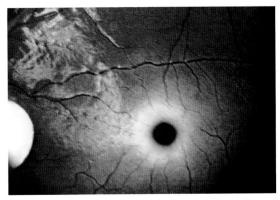

Fig. 5.2 Cherry-red spot in the fundus of an infant with Tay-Sachs disease. (From Taylor D, Hoyt CS 2005 Pediatric Ophthalmology and Strabismus, 3rd edn. Saunders, London.)

Section 6
Pediatric: Tumors

Rhabdomyosarcoma

Key Facts

- Most common primary orbital malignancy of childhood
- Malignant neoplasm of extraocular muscle precursor cells
- Age of diagnosis 7–8, with slight male predominance
- Associated nosebleed and sinusitis

Clinical Findings

- Sudden and rapid onset of proptosis
- Bruising around orbit
- Superior nasal orbital mass

Ancillary Testing

- Orbital biopsy with electron microscopy
- **MRI with contrast and fat suppression:**
  - irregular well-circumscribed mass
- **CAT scan:**
  - displays bone destruction
- Oncology evaluation with metastatic work-up

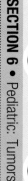
Differential Diagnosis

- Lymphangioma
- Hemangioma
- Orbital pseudotumor
- Orbital cellulitis
- Dermoid
- Neuroblastoma

Treatment

- Surgical resection of smaller well-circumscribed tumors or debulking of larger tumors
- Combination chemotherapy and external beam irradiation

Prognosis

- Depends on subtype, but 90% survival with isolated confined orbital lesions
- **Visual outcome depends on degree of:**
  - proptosis • corneal exposure • complications of radiation treatment (including retinopathy, keratoconjunctivitis sicca, optic atrophy)

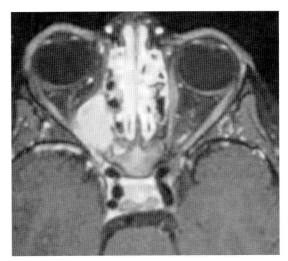

Fig. 6.1 Axial T₁ fat saturation MRI with gadolinium, showing enhancing intraorbital rhabdomysarcoma.

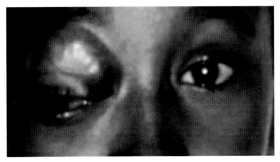

Fig. 6.2 Right superior intraorbital rhabdomysarcoma.

Neuroblastoma

Key Facts

- Orbital metastatic tumor seen in 20% of patients with neuroblastoma
- Originates from adrenal gland or sympathetic ganglion in retroperitoneum or mediastinum
- **Systemic symptoms include:**
  - abdominal distension • renal vascular hypertension • bone pain

Clinical Findings

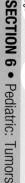

- **Orbital metastasis:**
  - proptosis • lid ecchymosis
- **Intrathoracic or sympathetic tumor:**
  - Horner syndrome
- **Paraneoplastic syndrome:**
  - opsoclonus (rapid, random, saccadic nystagmus)

Ancillary Testing

- Biopsy of lesion diagnostic
- Urine catecholamines positive in 90% of cases
- Abdominal ultrasound, CT scan, or MRI with full metastatic evaluation

Differential Diagnosis

- Lymphangioma
- Orbital dermoid or teratoma
- Rhabdomyosarcoma
- Hemangiopericytoma
- Rhabdomyosarcoma
- Burkitt lymphoma
- Optic glioma
- Sinus mucocele

Treatment

- Excision of isolated tumor
- Radiation and chemotherapy

Prognosis

- Prognosis worse with orbital involvement
- Opsoclonus without orbital involvement has better prognosis

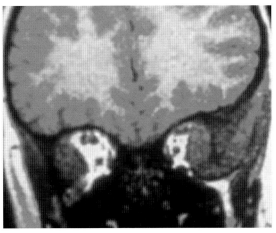

Fig. 6.3 Coronal MRI showing bilateral intraobital neuroblastoma.

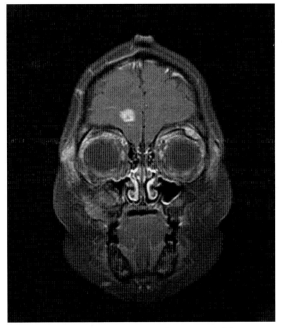

Fig. 6.4 Coronal T$_1$ fat saturation MRI with gadolinium, showing enhancing metastatic lesions to the left superotemporal orbital rim and frontal lobe.

Leukemia

Key Facts

- Ocular findings with acute lymphoblastic, acute myelogenous, and acute monocytic leukemia

Clinical Findings

- Flame-shaped retinal hemorrhages
- White-centered retinal hemorrhage
- Choroidal thickening
- Optic nerve swelling if leukemic infiltration
- Possible anterior segment leukemic infiltration with heterochromia iridis, keratic precipitates, spontaneous hyphema, and/or hypopyon
- Glaucoma may develop from tumor cells clogging trabecular meshwork or pupillary block from synechiae formation

Ancillary Testing

- Anterior chamber paracentesis for cytologic evaluation
- Systemic evaluation including white blood cell count and bone marrow aspiration
- B-scan ultrasound if choroidal involvement suspected

Differential Diagnosis

- **Intraretinal hemorrhages:**
  - anemia or other bleeding diathesis
  - disseminated endothelial infection (e.g. subacute bacterial endocarditis)
  - diabetes mellitus
- **Optic disc swelling:**
  - optic neuritis
  - autoimmune optic neuropathy (e.g. sarcoid)
  - infectious optic neuropathy (e.g. Lyme disease)
- **Anterior chamber inflammation or hyphema:**
  - juvenile rheumatoid arthritis
  - trauma
  - juvenile xanthogranuloma

Treatment

- Chemotherapy
- Radiation treatment if optic nerve involvement and infiltration

Prognosis

- Depends on extent of systemic and ocular involvement
- Typically poorer prognosis in children who have ocular involvement
- **Risk of complication from irradiation, including:**
  - cataract formation • radiation retinopathy • keratoconjunctivitis sicca • optic atrophy

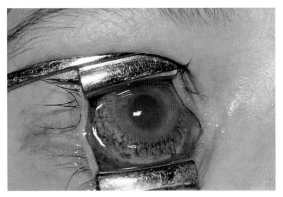

Fig. 6.5 Acute lymphoblastic leukemia with eye relapse presenting as an acute red and painful eye due to glaucoma. (From Taylor D, Hoyt CS 2005 Pediatric Ophthalmology and Strabismus, 3rd edn. Saunders, London.)

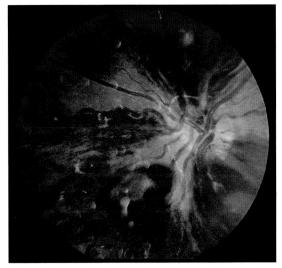

Fig. 6.6 Retinal hemorrhages and infiltrates in acute lymphoblastic leukemia. (From Taylor D, Hoyt CS 2005 Pediatric Ophthalmology and Strabismus, 3rd edn. Saunders, London.)

Capillary Hemangioma of the Lid and Orbit

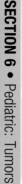

Key Facts

- Most common benign orbital tumors of childhood
- 2 : 1 female to male ratio
- Endothelial cell proliferation with small vascular channels on pathologic examination
- Typically enlarge rapidly during first few months of life, with maximum size reached by 1 year
- Spontaneous involution begins during second year of life
- Complete regression in 40% of cases by age 4, 80% by age 8 years
- **Kasabach–Merritt syndrome:**
  - thrombocytopenia secondary to platelet sequestration within large lesions
- Posterior fossa malformations, hemangioma, arterial anomalies, coarctation of the aorta, eye abnormalities, and sternum abnormalities (PHACES) syndrome

Clinical Findings

- **Upper eyelid involvement with ptosis:**
  - deprivational or occlusional amblyopia
  - astigmatism with anisometropic amblyopia
- **Variable orbital extension with proptosis:**
  - exposure keratitis
  - optic neuropathy

Ancillary Testing

- Full ophthalmic examination including retinoscopy
- Assessment of vision using visual evoked potential or preferential looking in preverbal children
- B-scan ultrasound, orbital CT or MRI to determine extent of orbital involvement
- Cardiac and neurologic evaluation if PHACES syndrome in consideration

Differential Diagnosis

- Lymphangioma
- Neuroblastoma
- Rhabdomyosarcoma
- Hemangiopericytoma
- Orbital dermoid
- Burkitt lymphoma
- Optic glioma
- Sinus mucocele

Treatment

- Intralesional corticosteroid injection
  - Risk of fat atrophy, skin depigmentation, or central retinal artery occlusion
- Oral corticosteroids (1–3 mg/kg per day prednisone or equivalent)
- Complete excision difficult, although partial excision may be required if limited response to corticoids and vision-threatening
- Treat resultant amblyopia if present with corrective lenses and occlusion therapy to good eye

Prognosis

- **Depends on extent of:**
  - ptosis • orbital involvement • subsequent complications
- Overall for smaller lesions excellent visual prognosis, because these lesions respond well to corticosteroids and regress spontaneously

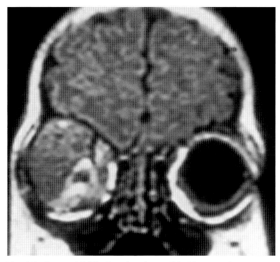
Fig. 6.7 Coronal MRI showing intraorbital hemangioma.

Lymphangioma

Key Facts

- Second most common orbital vascular tumor of childhood
- Small blood vessels with thin walls separate lymph-filled channels
- Hemorrhages spontaneously or after minor trauma
- Primarily orbital but may be localized to eyelid or conjunctiva

Clinical Findings

- Eyelid hematoma
- Subconjunctival hemorrhage
- Proptosis gradual with growth of lesion during first years of life
- Rapid proptosis with lymphoid hyperplasia secondary to upper respiratory tract infection, or intralesional bleeding chocolate cyst typically after 5 years of age

Ancillary Testing

- CT or MRI scan with gadolinium (variable enhancement of cyst)
- Biopsy can be performed, but risk of hemorrhage

Differential Diagnosis

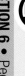

- Rhabdomyosarcoma
- Neuroblastoma
- Leukemia
- Capillary hemangioma
- Dermoid
- Teratoma
- Sarcoma
- Glioma

Treatment

- **Medical management:**
  - restrict activity
  - cold compress
  - treat corneal exposure if present
- **Surgical management:**
  - evacuation of cyst if optic neuropathy develops
  - carbon dioxide laser can be used to debulk lesion

Prognosis

- Depends on extent of proptosis and optic neuropathy

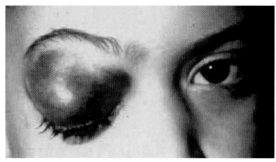

Fig. 6.8 Lymphangioma involving the right upper lid and orbit.

Orbital Dermoid Cyst

Key Facts

- Most common benign orbital space–occupying lesion of childhood
- Choristoma comprising normal cell and tissue types not typically found at this location
- **Keratinized epithelial cyst with dermal appendages:**
  - hair follicles • sebaceous glands • sweat glands
- Occurs at fetal suture line, most commonly superotemporal or superonasal
- Typically of no visual consequence

Clinical Findings

- Smooth, non-tender mass that is often immobile if attached to bone at suture line
- Small ruptures of cyst wall can occur, leading to excessive inflammation and mild tenderness

Ancillary Testing

- **CT scan:**
  - bony remodeling or defect can occur

Differential Diagnosis

- Lymphangioma
- Neuroblastoma
- Rhabdomyosarcoma
- Hemangiopericytoma
- Rhabdomyosarcoma
- Burkitt lymphoma
- Optic glioma
- Sinus mucocele or meningoencephalocele

Treatment

- **Surgical excision:**
  - avoid rupture of cyst, because this can lead to an aggressive inflammatory reaction
  - if unable to remove in total and cyst ruptures, irrigate and remove cyst lining to limit recurrence

Prognosis

- Excellent if able to be removed completely with cyst lining intact
- Lipogranulomatous inflammation and scarring can occur if cyst ruptures

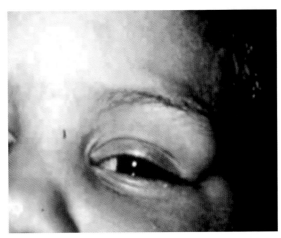
Fig. 6.9 Dermoid cyst involving left superotemporal orbital rim at the zygomatic-frontal suture.

Teratoma

Key Facts

- Choristoma containing multiple tissues derived from all three germinal layers (ectoderm, mesoderm, endoderm)
  - Most common: skin and dermal appendages, neural tissue, muscle, and bone
  - Less common: respiratory and gastrointestinal tract epithelium
- Extensive proptosis can cause optic neuropathy

Clinical Findings

- Partially cystic intraorbital lesion
- Proptosis

Ancillary Testing

- **CT scan:**
  - bony remodeling or defect can occur

Differential Diagnosis

- Lymphangioma
- Neuroblastoma
- Rhabdomyosarcoma
- Hemangiopericytoma
- Rhabdomyosarcoma
- Burkitt lymphoma
- Optic glioma
- Sinus mucocele

Treatment

- **Surgical excision:**
  - prior aspiration of fluid sometimes necessary

Prognosis

- Depends on ease of surgical excision and extent of optic neuropathy if present

SECTION 6 • Pediatric: Tumors

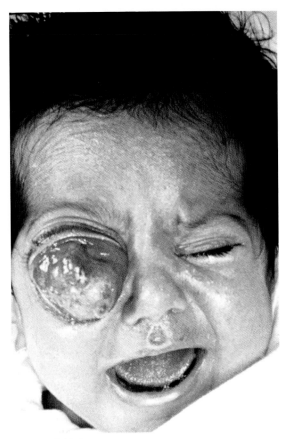

Fig. 6.10 Orbital teratoma.

Retinoblastoma

Key Facts

- Neuroblastic tumor arising from retinal photoreceptor precursor cells
- 50% sporadic with 50% hereditary (autosomal dominant), although <25% have family history
- Occurs in 1 in 15000 births
- Tumor develops because of deletion of both cellular copies of Rb gene (a tumor suppressor gene)
- Bilaterality and multifocal lesions often seen in hereditary cases
- Average age of diagnosis 1 year for hereditary cases, 2 years for sporadic cases
- Rare presentation after age 5

Clinical Findings

- Leukocoria
- Visual inattentiveness
- Strabismus
- Orbital cellulitis-like picture in advanced cases with tumor necrosis and inflammation
- White or cream-colored mass involving vitreous and retina
- Vitreous seeding
- Pineoblastoma (trilateral retinoblastoma)
- Pseudohypopyon of tumor cells

Ancillary Testing

- **CT scan:**
  - calcifications present within lesion
  - can rule out pineoblastoma
- MRI may be preferable to lessen radiation-induced risk of secondary tumors in hereditary cases
- B-scan ultrasound shows mass with possible intralesional calcifications and retinal detachment

Differential Diagnosis

- Coats disease
- Norrie disease
- Toxoplasmosis
- *Toxocara canis*
- Familial exudative vitreoretinpopathy
- Persistent fetal vasculature
- Pars planitis
- Retinal astrocytoma
- Cataract

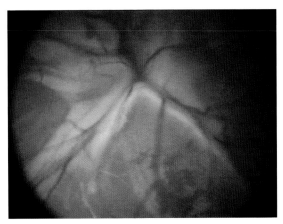

Fig. 6.11 Unilateral exophytic retinoblastoma with retinal detachment. (From Taylor D, Hoyt CS 2005 Pediatric Ophthalmology and Strabismus, 3rd edn. Saunders, London.)

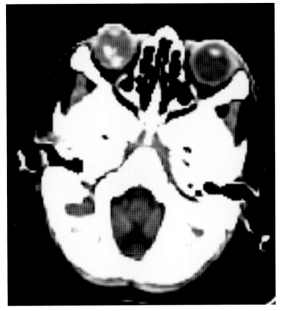

Fig. 6.12 CT scan of exophytic retinoblastoma, showing intraocular calcium. (From Taylor D, Hoyt CS 2005 Pediatric Ophthalmology and Strabismus, 3rd edn. Saunders, London.)

Treatment

- **Depends on:**
  - size • number of tumors • location of tumors • bilaterality
- **Includes:**
  - chemoreduction • cryotherapy • laser ablation • plaque or external beam radiation • enucleation

Prognosis

- Mortality 100% if untreated
- >90% survival rate if treated
- Risk of complication from irradiation, including secondary tumors (especially osteosarcoma)
- **Risk of:**
  - cataract formation • radiation retinopathy • keratoconjunctivitis sicca • optic atrophy

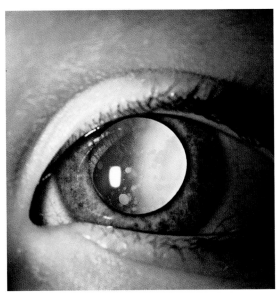

Fig. 6.13 External photograph of endophytic retinoblastoma with vitreous seeds. (Courtesy of IIRC Group E.)

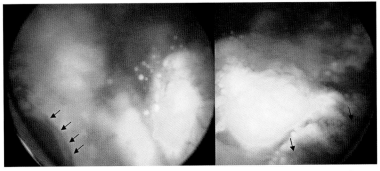

Fig. 6.14 Retinal photograph of endophytic retinoblastoma with vitreous seeding with extension to the ora serrata (arrows). (From Taylor D, Hoyt CS 2005 Pediatric Ophthalmology and Strabismus, 3rd edn. Saunders, London.)

Section 7

Pediatric: Phakomatoses

Neurofibromatosis (von Recklinghausen Disease)

Key Facts

- Genetically predisposed hamartoma composed of melanocytes or neuroglial cells of neural crest origin
- Prevalence of 1 in 3000–5000
- Predominantly autosomal dominant but can be sporadic
- **Neurofibromatosis (NF) type 1:**
  - long arm of chromosome 17
  - more common than NF type 2
  - café-au-lait spots (six or more >5 mm in diameter in prepubescents, >15 mm in postpubescents)
  - axillary or inguinal freckling
  - nodular cutaneous and subcutaneous neurofibromas
  - sphenoid bone dysplasia or thinning of long bone complex
- **NF type 2:**
  - long arm of chromosome 22
  - meningioma and schwannoma

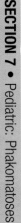

Clinical Findings

- **NF type 1:**
  - plexiform neurofibroma
  - iris Lisch's nodules
  - optic nerve glioma
  - prominent corneal nerves
  - retinal hamartomas
  - glaucoma, strabismus, and amblyopia
- **NF type 2:**
  - iris Lisch's nodules
  - combined hamartoma of retina and retinal pigment epithelium
  - posterior subcapsular cataract
  - optic nerve glioma

Ancillary Testing

- Visual fields and color vision testing
- MRI scan of brain
- Genetic evaluation

Differential Diagnosis

- Tuberous sclerosis
- von Hippel–Lindau syndrome
- Sturge–Weber syndrome
- Ataxia-telangiectasia
- Racemose angioma

Treatment

- Treat associated amblyopia, glaucoma, and cataract
- Debulk plexiform neurofibroma if visually significant
- Monitor for development of optic nerve glioma with appropriate referral for treatment

Prognosis

- Depends on extent of ocular findings, especially glaucoma, cataract, and optic nerve glioma
- Lisch's nodules visually insignificant

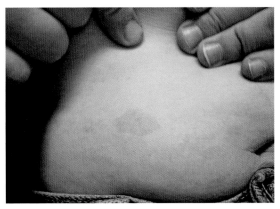

Fig. 7.1 Café-au-lait spot in neurofibromatosis.

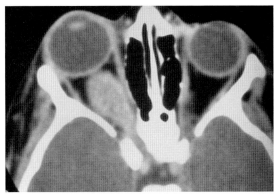

Fig. 7.2 Axial CT showing optic nerve glioma.

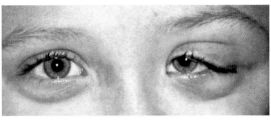

Fig. 7.3 Left upper lid plexiform neurofibroma in neurofibromatosis.

Lisch's Nodules

Key Facts

- Hamartomas of iris associated with neurofibromatosis type 1
- Neural crest origin
- Histology shows focal aggregates of melanocytes and glial cells on anterior border layer of iris
- Prevalence in neurofibromatosis patients is approximately 10 times the patient's age

Clinical Findings

- Discrete, multiple, lightly pigmented nodules
- **Other ocular manifestations of neurofibromatosis type 1:**
  - plexiform neurofibroma of eyelid and orbit • glaucoma • choroidal hamartoma • schwannoma • optic nerve pilocytic astrocytoma (glioma)

Ancillary Testing

- Dermatologic evaluation for café-au-lait spots

Differential Diagnosis

- Juvenile xanthogranuloma
- Iris cysts

Treatment

- None required

Prognosis

- Lisch's nodules visually insignificant
- Overall visual prognosis depends on extent of other ocular findings in neurofibromatosis

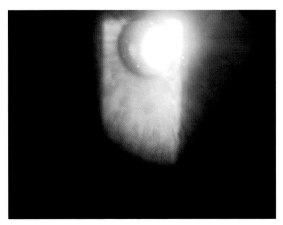

Fig. 7.4 Multiple iris Lisch's nodules.

Tuberous Sclerosis (Bourneville Disease)

Key Facts

- **Benign tumor growth in multiple organ systems:**
  - skin • brain • heart • kidney • eye
- Prevalence of 1 in 10 000
- Autosomal dominant with incomplete penetrance and spontaneous mutations
  - Tuberous sclerosis type 1: 9q34
  - Tuberous sclerosis type 2: 16p13.3
- **Vogt triad:**
  - mental retardation • seizures • facial angiofibromas
- **Adenoma sebaceum:** facial angiofibroma
- **Shagreen patch:** thickened skin plaque
- **Ash leaf sign:** depigmented skin macule
- Subungual fibromas
- **Subependymal and cortical astrocytomas:**
  - can calcify potato-like masses • cortical tuber
- Renal lesions and cardiac rhabdomyomas

Clinical Findings

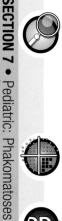

- **Astrocytic hamartoma of retina:**
  - gray-white, flat, smooth surface, indistinct margins, typically in younger children
  - sharply demarcated, opaque, yellow-white, calcified, elevated, irregular surface (like tapioca or fish eggs)
- Astrocytic hamartoma of optic nerve (giant drusen)
- Rare cases of neovascular glaucoma and retinal detachment
- 40% bilateral

Ancillary Testing

- Fluorescein angiography
- MRI or CT scan of brain
- Neurologic, renal, and cardiac evaluation

Differential Diagnosis

- Neurofibromatosis
- von Hippel–Lindau syndrome
- Sturge–Weber syndrome
- Ataxia-telangiectasia
- Racemose angioma

Treatment

- Treat strabismus and amblyopia if present
- Treat any associated retinal detachment

Prognosis

- Typically asymptomatic, non-progressive, with excellent visual prognosis, but may depend on location of astrocytoma and optic nerve involvement

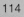

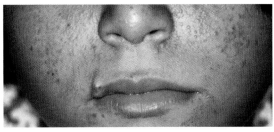

Fig. 7.5 Angiofibroma involving the upper lip in tuberous sclerosis.

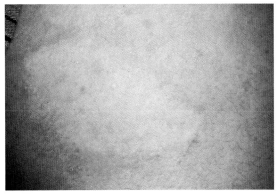

Fig. 7.6 Ash leaf sign in tuberous sclerosis.

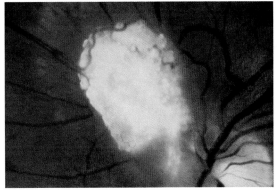

Fig. 7.7 Astrocytic hamartoma extending off the optic nerve in tuberous sclerosis.

Tuberous Sclerosis (Bourneville Disease) (Continued)

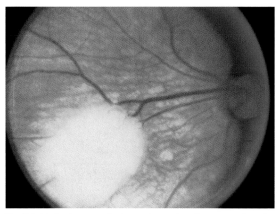

Fig. 7.8 Retinal astrocytic hamartoma in tuberous sclerosis.

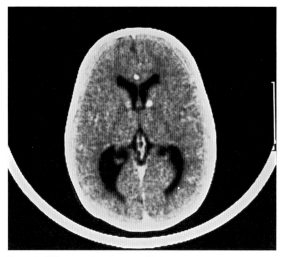

Fig. 7.9 CT scan showing calcified cortical astrocytoma in tuberous sclerosis.

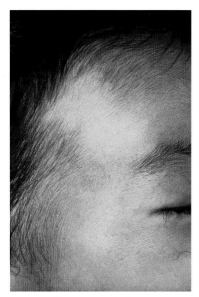

Fig. 7.10 Shagreen patch in tuberous sclerosis.

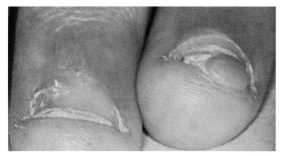

Fig. 7.11 Subungual fibroma in tuberous sclerosis.

von Hippel–Lindau Syndrome (Retinal Angiomatosis)

Key Facts

- Benign and malignant capillary hemangioma tumor growth in multiple organ systems
- Prevalence of 1 in 36 000
- **Autosomal dominant:**
  - partial deletion of tumor suppressor gene on chromosome 3
- No major cutaneous involvement
- Cerebellar hemangioblastoma
- Renal cell carcinoma, pheochromocytoma, renal and pancreatic cysts
- von Hippel described the retinal angiomas and Lindau the cerebellar lesions

Clinical Findings

- Capillary hemangioma of retina or optic nerve
  - Often multiple and bilateral
  - Dilated tortuous afferent artery and efferent vein
- May develop retinal detachment and gliosis secondary to transudation of fluid into subretinal space

Ancillary Testing

- **Fluorescein angiography:**
  - tumor fills rapidly during arterial phase • marked hyperfluorescence in venous phase • dye leakage in late phase
- MRI or CT scan of brain, with attention to cerebellum
- Neurologic evaluation
- Renal ultrasound
- 24-h urine for vanillylmandelic acids
- Genetic evaluation

Differential Diagnosis

- Neurofibromatosis
- Tuberous sclerosis
- Sturge–Weber syndrome
- Ataxia-telangiectasia
- Racemose angioma

Treatment

- Treat strabismus and amblyopia if present
- No treatment required for small asymptomatic non-leaking retinal tumors
- Argon laser, cryotherapy, or photodynamic therapy if tumor grows with accumulation of exudation or subretinal fluid
  - Smaller lesions easier to treat
- Optic nerve tumors notoriously difficult to treat without severe visual loss
- Treat any associated retinal detachment

Prognosis

- Small retinal tumors typically asymptomatic initially, remain stable, and can even regress spontaneously
- Larger tumors may lead to severe visual loss if significant subretinal fluid, exudation, or retinal detachment occurs

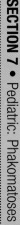

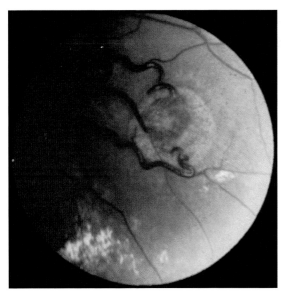

Fig. 7.12 Capillary hemangioma of the retina in von Hippel–
Lindau syndrome.

Sturge–Weber Syndrome (Encephalofacial Angiomatosis)

Key Facts

- No hereditary transmission
- Lesions present at birth
- **Cutaneous angioma (also called nevus flammeus or port wine stain):**
  - typically involves forehead and upper eyelid
  - may involve trunk and extremities
  - hypertrophy of soft tissue and bone underlying angioma (Klippel–Trenaunay–Weber syndrome)
- **Ipsilateral leptomeningeal hemangioma:**
  - most pronounced in occipital region
  - calcification of adjacent cerebral cortex (railroad track sign)
  - focal neurologic defects
  - seizures

Clinical Findings

- Increased conjunctival vascularity
- Choroidal angiomatosis (diffuse tomato catsup appearance)
  - Choroidal thickening or retinal detachment may occur
- **Glaucoma:**
  - secondary to presumed increased episcleral venous pressure, ciliary body hypersecretion, or developmental angle abnormality
  - upper lid angioma increases risk
  - buphthalmos may occur if onset of glaucoma in infancy

Ancillary Testing

- MRI or CT scan of brain
- Neurologic evaluation

Differential Diagnosis

- Neurofibromatosis
- Tuberous sclerosis
- von Hippel–Lindau syndrome
- Ataxia-telangiectasia
- Racemose angioma

Treatment

- Treat strabismus and amblyopia if present
- Pulsed dye laser for cutaneous angioma
- No effective treatment of choroidal angioma
- Laser photocoagulation, cryotherapy, or irradiation for secondary retinal detachment
- Treat glaucoma if present, although IOP difficult to regulate
  - Aqueous shunting devices typically necessary

Prognosis

- Depends on extent of glaucoma and complications from retinal angiomatosis

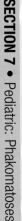

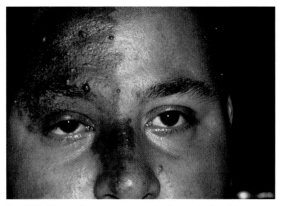
Fig. 7.13 Nevus flammeus or port wine stain involving forehead and upper eyelid in Sturge–Weber syndrome.

Ataxia-telangiectasia

Key Facts

- Autosomal recessive
- Abnormality in genes on chromosome 11
  - Women heterozygotes at high risk for breast cancer
- Prevalence of 1 in 40 000
- **Cerebellar involvement:**
  - progressive ataxia in childhood
  - progresses to dysarthria, dystonia, and choreoathetosis by age 10
- **Defective T-cell function with thymic hypoplasia:**
  - recurrent respiratory tract infections
  - increased incidence of lymphoma and leukemia

Clinical Findings

- Inability to initiate saccades similar to oculomotor apraxia
- Strabismus and nystagmus often present
- Conjunctival telangectasia develops by age 5
  - Initially interpalpebral then becoming generalized

Ancillary Testing

- MRI or CT scan of brain
- Neurologic and genetic evaluation

Differential Diagnosis

- Sturge–Weber syndrome
- Racemose angioma

Treatment

- Treat strabismus and amblyopia if present
- Appropriate treatment of secondary infections

Prognosis

- Early mortality secondary to recurrent infections, leukemia, or lymphoma

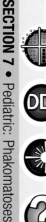

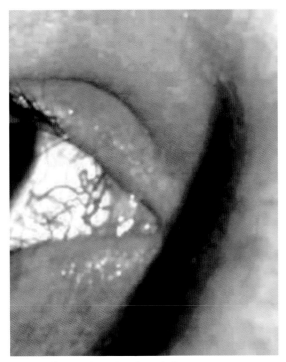

Fig. 7.14 Conjunctival telangiectasia in ataxia-telangiectasia.

Racemose Angioma (Wyburn–Mason Syndrome)

Key Facts

- Non-hereditary
- **Arteriovenous malformation of midbrain:**
  - seizures and focal neurologic defects
  - intracranial hemorrhage
- Occasional skin lesions may be present, facial hemangioma

Clinical Findings

- Arteriovenous malformation involving optic disc or retina
- Primarily unilateral
- Possible intraocular hemorrhage and secondary neovascular glaucoma

Ancillary Testing

- Fluorescein angiography
- MRI or CT scan of brain
- Neurologic evaluation

Differential Diagnosis

- von Hippel–Lindau syndrome
- Sturge–Weber syndrome
- Ataxia-telangiectasia

Treatment

- Treat strabismus and amblyopia if present
- Treat glaucoma with panretinal photocoagulation
- Vitrectomy if persistent intraocular hemorrhage develops

Prognosis

- Visual involvement depends on size and location of retinal racemose hemangioma

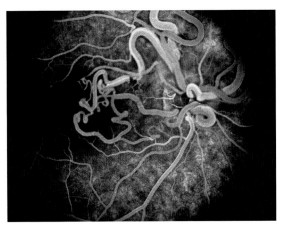

Fig. 7.15 Fluorescein angiogram of racemose angioma.

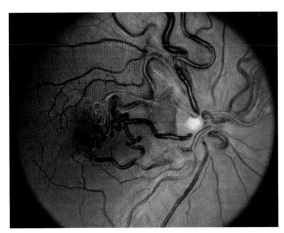

Fig. 7.16 Retinal photograph of racemose angioma.

Section 8

Pediatric:
Craniosynostosis

Crouzon Syndrome

Key Facts

- Premature closure of one or more of the metopic, sagittal, or lambdoidal sutures
  • Skull brachycephaly from bilateral coronal suture closure • Midface hypoplasia and malocclusion • Hearing impairment and mental retardation may be present

Clinical Findings

- Shallow orbit with proptosis
  • Corneal exposure • Possible globe prolapse with optic neuropathy
- Exophthalmos • V-pattern exotropia exacerbated by orbital excyclotorsion and rectus muscle displacement • Possible amblyopia • Associated aniridia, iris coloboma, microcornea, megalocornea, cataract, ectopia lentis, and glaucoma

Ancillary Testing

- CT or MRI of head and orbits

Differential Diagnosis

- Apert syndrome • Pfeiffer syndrome

Treatment

- Treat corneal exposure • Possible tarsorrhaphy if globe prolapse • Repair strabismus and any associated amblyopia • Multidisciplinary cranial–facial reconstruction

Prognosis

- Depends on degree of proptosis with corneal exposure and optic neuropathy

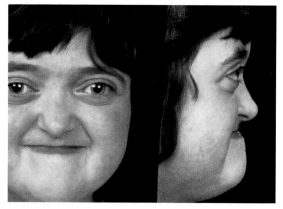

Fig. 8.1 This girl has the features of inferior prognathism, maxillary hypoplasia, and a prominent forehead, while her nose is quite straight—it is more "hooked" in this condition. (From Taylor D, Hoyt CS 2005 Pediatric Ophthalmology and Strabismus, 3rd edn. Saunders, London.)

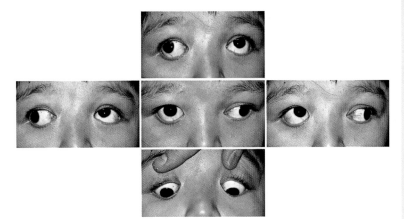

Fig. 8.2 V-pattern esotropia characteristic of Crouzon syndrome, Apert syndrome, and other craniofacial syndromes. (From Taylor D, Hoyt CS 2005 Pediatric Ophthalmology and Strabismus, 3rd edn. Saunders, London.)

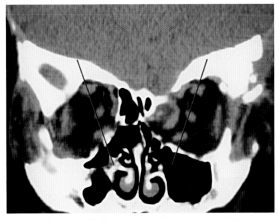

Fig. 8.3 Coronal CT showing extorsion of both orbits and their contents, which has been emphasized by lines drawn between the centers of the superior and inferior rectus muscles on each side. (From Taylor D, Hoyt CS 2005 Pediatric Ophthalmology and Strabismus, 3rd edn. Saunders, London.)

Apert Syndrome

Key Facts

- Premature closure of midline structures secondary to cartilage dysplasia at cranial base • Skull brachycephaly from bilateral coronal suture closure • Cerebral malformations including ventriculomegaly • Deficient supraorbital ridge replaced by a horizontal groove and midface hypoplasia with upward tilting • Symmetric hand and feet syndactyly with nail fusion • Elbow and shoulder joint abnormalities • Mental retardation may be present

Clinical Findings

- Shallow orbit with proptosis (often less marked than in Crouzon syndrome) • Corneal exposure • Possible globe prolapse with optic neuropathy
- Exophthalmos • V-pattern exotropia exacerbated by orbital excyclotorsion and rectus muscle displacement • Possible amblyopia • Associated keratoconus, ectopia lentis, and glaucoma

Ancillary Testing

- CT or MRI of head and orbits

Differential Diagnosis

- Crouzon syndrome • Pfeiffer syndrome

Treatment

- Treat corneal exposure • Possible tarsorrhaphy if globe prolapse • Repair strabismus and any associated amblyopia • Multidisciplinary cranial–facial reconstruction

Prognosis

- Depends on degree of proptosis with corneal exposure and optic neuropathy

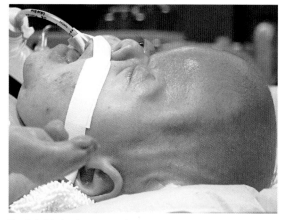

Fig. 8.4 Marked asymmetric proptosis in Apert syndrome, with recurrent spontaneous globe luxation and hypoplasia of the brow and maxilla. (From Taylor D, Hoyt CS 2005 Pediatric Ophthalmology and Strabismus, 3rd edn. Saunders, London.)

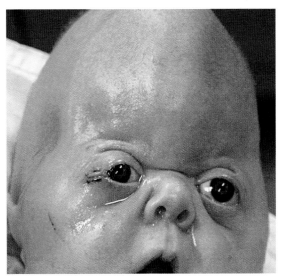

Fig. 8.5 Lateral tarsorrhaphy in Apert syndrome to prevent globe luxation. (From Taylor D, Hoyt CS 2005 Pediatric Ophthalmology and Strabismus, 3rd edn. Saunders, London.)

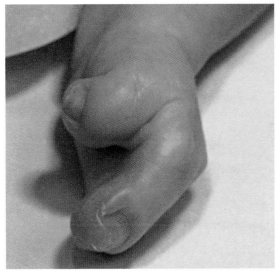

Fig. 8.6 Symmetric syndactyly affecting the second to fifth digits of the hands and feet with nail fusion in Apert syndrome. (From Taylor D, Hoyt CS 2005 Pediatric Ophthalmology and Strabismus, 3rd edn. Saunders, London.)

Section 9
Pediatric: Other Disorders

Fetal Alcohol Syndrome

Key Facts

- Alcohol-related neurodevelopmental disorder, alcohol-related birth defects, fetal alcohol spectrum disorders
- Malformations seen in children born to women with a history of heavy alcohol use during pregnancy
- Extent of defects depends on consumption, timing, and genetics
- Reduced birth length and weight
- Long, flat, smooth philtrum
- Thin vermilion border
- Anteverted nostrils
- Abnormal corpus callosum, cerebellum, or basal ganglia
- Cardiovascular, urogenital, and skeletal abnormalities
- Global cognitive or intellectual deficits

Clinical Findings

- Asymmetric ptosis
- Small palpebral fissure
- Strabismus and amblyopia
- Anterior segment dysgenesis
- Optic nerve hypoplasia
- Retinal vascular tortuosity

Ancillary Testing

- Neurologic, educational, and social service referral
- MRI of brain

Differential Diagnosis

- Craniosynostosis
- Trisomy 21
- Williams syndrome

Treatment

- Treat associated strabismus and amblyopia
- Ptosis repair if visually significant
- Neuropsychologic assessment and treatment

Prognosis

- Depends on extent of central nervous system and optic nerve involvement
- Depends on degree of and response to treatment for ptosis, strabismus, and amblyopia

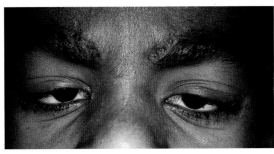
Fig. 9.1 Small palpebral fissures in fetal alcohol syndrome.

Shaken Baby Syndrome

Key Facts

- Non-accidental trauma with multisystem injury, especially intracranial, ocular, and skeletal
- Primarily in children <3 years old with poor neck stabilization
- Often history by caregiver of minor trauma that is inconsistent with degree of injuries
- Occurs in children of all socioeconomic backgrounds
- Not caused by cardiopulmonary resuscitation
- **Intracranial injury:** subdural or subarachnoid hemorrhage secondary to rupture of bridging vessels from abrupt repetitive acceleration then deceleration of brain within cranium
- Ocular findings usually bilateral but may be unilateral

Clinical Findings

- Vitreous hemorrhage
- Preretinal hemorrhages
- Hemorrhage in multiple retinal layers of different configurations (dot blot, flame-shaped, white-centered)
  - No specific pathognomonic lesion
- Full-thickness retinal folding
- Hemorrhage and folding typically involves the macula
- Retinoschisis

Ancillary Testing

- MRI of brain
- X-rays of long bones for evidence of prior fractures or abuse
- Hematologic evaluation to rule out a clotting disorder
- Social service referral, notification of appropriate authorities for child protection
- Physician may have a legal obligation to report case to appropriate authorities

Differential Diagnosis

- Birth trauma
- Accidental trauma
- Bleeding disorder

Treatment

- Vitrectomy for vitreous hemorrhage if persistent and visually significant
- Treat associated amblyopia or strabismus
- Remove child from at-risk environment

Prognosis

- Depends on extent of central nervous system, optic nerve, and retinal involvement
- Overall mortality rate of approximately 25%
- Survivors often have permanent neurologic and visual impairment

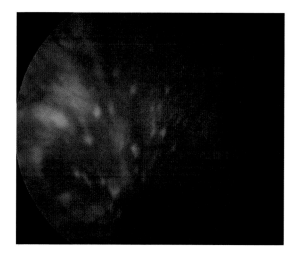

Fig. 9.2 Diffuse intraretinal hemorrhage and white-centered hemorrhages in shaken baby syndrome.

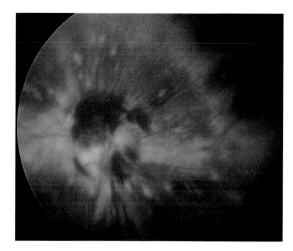

Fig. 9.3 Hemorrhagic papilledema, flame-shaped hemorrhages, and intraretinal white-centered hemorrhages in shaken baby syndrome.

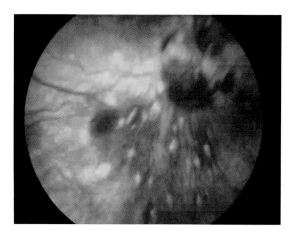

Fig. 9.4 Subhyaloid and intravitreal hemorrhage in shaken baby syndrome.

Section

10

Strabismus: Esodeviations

Pseudoesotropia

Key Facts

- With visual axis aligned, there is a false appearance of esotropia
- Common cause of infant referral to an ophthalmologist

Clinical Findings

- Flat, broad nasal bridge
- Prominent epicanthal folds
- Narrow interpupillary distance
- Normal corneal light reflex
- No movement on cover–uncover test

Ancillary Testing

- Cover testing
- Hirschberg or Krimsky light reflex test if unable to perform cover test
- Full ophthalmic examination including slit lamp and fundus

Differential Diagnosis

- Congenital esotropia
- Accommodative esotropia
- High AC : A ratio esotropia
- Divergence insufficiency
- Spasm of near reflex
- Consecutive esotropia
- **Non-comitant strabismus, i.e.:**
  - Duane syndrome type 1 • sixth nerve palsy • ocular myasthenia gravis
    - progressive external ophthalmoplegia • restrictive strabismus

Treatment

- None required

Prognosis

- With growth, epicanthal folds displace and the bridge of the nose becomes more prominent, decreasing the appearance of pseudoesotropia

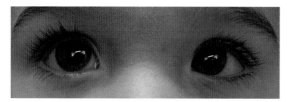
Fig. 10.1 Pseudoesotropia.

Congenital Esotropia

Key Facts
- Constant esotropia present before 6 months of age
- Often hereditary
- 1–2% incidence

Clinical Findings
- Cross-fixation or alternate fixation common
- Usually equal visual acuity, although amblyopia may be present
- Esotropia typically >30 PD
- Full abduction unless secondary medial rectus restriction
- Associated latent nystagmus, inferior oblique over-action, and dissociated vertical deviation

Ancillary Testing
- Cover–uncover and alternate cover testing
- Hirschberg or Krimsky light reflex test if unable to perform cover test
- Stereopsis testing
- Intraoperative forced duction testing to rule out secondary medial rectus restriction

Differential Diagnosis
- Pseudoesotropia
- Accommodative esotropia
- High AC : A ratio esotropia
- Divergence insufficiency
- Spasm of near reflex
- Consecutive esotropia
- **Non-comitant strabismus, i.e.:**
  - Duane syndrome type 1 • sixth nerve palsy • ocular myasthenia gravis • progressive external ophthalmoplegia • restrictive strabismus

Treatment
- Treat significant refractive error and amblyopia if present with spectacles and occlusion therapy
- **Surgery:** align to within 8 PD of orthotropia
  - Ability to develop stereopsis increases if performed before 1 year of age
  - Bilateral medial rectus recessions
  - Bilateral lateral rectus resections
  - Uniocular medial rectus recession and lateral rectus resection

Prognosis
- Excellent visual prognosis if early surgery and compliant with amblyopia treatment
- Variable development of stereopsis

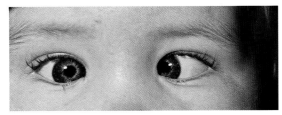

Fig. 10.2 Congenital esotropia. (From Taylor D, Hoyt CS 2005 Pediatric Ophthalmology and Strabismus, 3rd edn. Saunders, London.)

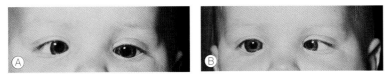

Fig. 10.3 Cross-fixation in congenital esotropia (**A**) The left eye is fixing the target and the right eye is deviating inwards. (**B**) Fixation is reversed spontaneously. (From Taylor D, Hoyt CS 2005 Pediatric Ophthalmology and Strabismus, 3rd edn. Saunders, London.)

Congenital Esotropia

Accommodative Esotropia

Key Facts

- **Alternative name:** refractive accommodative esotropia
- Accommodation from uncorrected hyperopia leads to excess convergence that overcomes fusional divergence
- Age of onset between 6 months and 7 years (average 2.5 years)
- Intermittent at onset then becoming constant
- Often hereditary
- Can be precipitated by illness or trauma

Clinical Findings

- Comitant esotropia typically 20–30 PD
- Average hyperopia of +4.00 D
- Amblyopia and reduced stereopsis may be present
- Diplopia may be present initially until image becomes suppressed

Ancillary Testing

- Cycloplegic retinoscopy with cyclopentolate or atropine drops necessary to determine full amount of hyperopia
- Cover–uncover and alternate cover testing
- Hirschberg or Krimsky light reflex test if unable to perform cover test
- Stereopsis testing

Differential Diagnosis

- Pseudoesotropia
- Congenital esotropia
- High AC : A ratio esotropia
- Divergence insufficiency
- Spasm of near reflex
- Consecutive esotropia
- **Non-comitant strabismus, i.e.:**
    - Duane syndrome type 1 • sixth nerve palsy • ocular myasthenia gravis
        - progressive external ophthalmoplegia • restrictive strabismus

Treatment

- Fully correct hyperopic refractive error determined by cycloplegic retinoscopy with spectacles or contact lenses
- Child must wear glasses full time
- Anticholinesterase drops may be tried if non-compliant with glasses
    - May cause iris cysts, and systemic absorption may interfere with general anesthesia
    - Concomitant use of phenylephrine to help prevent cysts
    - More susceptible to depolarizing agents because of lower pseudocholinesterase levels
- Occlusion therapy if amblyopia present
- Strabismus surgery may be required if residual esotropia despite hyperopia fully corrected and compliant with wearing spectacles

Prognosis

- Excellent visual prognosis if treated early and compliant with spectacles and occlusion therapy for amblyopia, if present

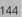

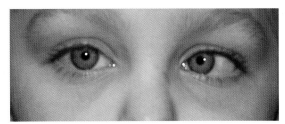

Fig. 10.4 Accommodative esotropia without glasses.

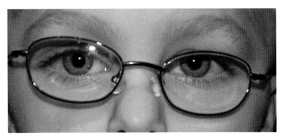

Fig. 10.5 Eyes straighten with hyperopic correction in accommodation esotropia.

High AC:A Ratio Esotropia

Key Facts

- **Alternative name:** non-refractive accommodative esotropia
- Esotropia develops because of abnormal relationship between accommodation and accommodative convergence (AC:A ratio)
- During near accommodation, excess convergence tonus leads to esotropia in setting of insufficient fusional divergence

Clinical Findings

- Esotropia greater at near than distance
- Esotropia reduced at near with a +3.00 D lens
- **Distance refraction can be:**
  - hyperopic (average +2.25 D) • myopic • emmetropic
- Reduced near stereopsis
- Amblyopia may be present

Ancillary Testing

- Cycloplegic retinoscopy with cyclopentolate or atropine drops necessary to determine full amount of hyperopia
- Cover–uncover and alternate cover testing at both distance and near with accommodative target
  - Remeasurement at near with full distance correction and additional +3.00 D correction
- Hirschberg or Krimsky light reflex test if unable to perform cover test
- Stereopsis testing

Differential Diagnosis

- Pseudoesotropia
- Congenital esotropia
- Accommodative esotropia
- Divergence insufficiency
- Spasm of near reflex
- Consecutive esotropia
- **Non-comitant strabismus, i.e.:**
  - Duane syndrome type 1 • sixth nerve palsy • ocular myasthenia gravis
    • progressive external ophthalmoplegia • restrictive strabismus

Treatment

- Fully correct refractive error determined by cycloplegic retinoscopy
- **Prescribe bifocals:** +2.50 to +3.00
  - Depends on alignment at preferred near reading distance
- Child must wear glasses full time
- Anticholinesterase drops may be tried
  - May cause iris cysts, and systemic absorption may interfere with general anesthesia
  - Concomitant use of phenylephrine to help prevent cysts
  - More susceptible to depolarizing agents because of lower pseudocholinesterase levels
- Occlusion therapy if amblyopia present
- Strabismus surgery controversial
- Monitor at least yearly, because bifocal reductions may be possible with advanced age

Prognosis

- Excellent visual prognosis if treated early and compliant with spectacles and occlusion therapy for amblyopia, if present

Divergence Insufficiency Esotropia

Key Facts

- More common in adults
- Deviation worse at distance than near
- Reduced fusional divergence
- **May be isolated or associated with underlying neurologic abnormality:**
  - head trauma • Parkinson disease • pontine lesion
- May complain of diplopia at distance

Clinical Findings

- Comitant esotropia greater at distance than near
- Full abduction

Ancillary Testing

- Cover–uncover and alternate cover testing at both distance and near
- Maddox rod, Hirschberg, or Krimsky light reflex test if unable to perform cover test
- CT or MRI scan of brain with contrast
- Full neurologic evaluation

Differential Diagnosis

- Pseudoesotropia
- Congenital esotropia
- Accommodative esotropia
- High AC:A ratio esotropia
- Spasm of near reflex
- Consecutive esotropia
- **Non-comitant strabismus, i.e.:**
  - Duane syndrome type 1 • sixth nerve palsy • ocular myasthenia gravis
    - progressive external ophthalmoplegia • restrictive strabismus

Treatment

- Base out prisms in distance correction to alleviate diplopia
- Strabismus surgery may be required
- Treat underlying neurologic condition if present

Prognosis

- Isolated divergence insufficiency may resolve
- Depends on ability to treat underlying neurologic condition

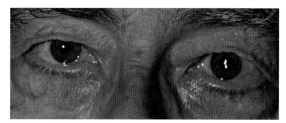

Fig. 10.6 Divergence insufficiency.

Spasm of the Near Reflex

Key Facts

- Abnormality of near response
- Usually functional
- May have underlying neurologic disease

Clinical Findings

- Esotropia with excessive accommodation and convergence
- Miosis
- Normal ductions with limited lateral gaze on version testing
- Myopic shift

Ancillary Testing

- Cover–uncover and alternate cover testing at both distance and near
- Hirschberg or Krimsky light reflex test if unable to perform cover test
- Cycloplegic retinoscopy
- Neurologic evaluation

Differential Diagnosis

- Pseudoesotropia
- Congenital esotropia
- Accommodative esotropia
- High AC : A ratio esotropia
- Divergence insufficiency
- Consecutive esotropia
- **Non-comitant strabismus, i.e.:**
  - Duane syndrome type 1 • sixth nerve palsy • ocular myasthenia gravis
    • progressive external ophthalmoplegia • restrictive strabismus

Treatment

- Fully correct any hyperopia
- Consider bifocals
- **Cycloplegic agents:** homatropine or atropine
- Treat underlying neurologic condition if present

Prognosis

- Problematic
- Depends on ability to treat underlying neurologic condition

Consecutive Esotropia

Key Facts

- Convergent strabismus after treatment of exotropia
- Esotropia from slipped or stretched muscle after exotropia surgery
- Esotropia from inability to establish fusion after surgical alignment of exotropia
- Can occur acutely or years later

Clinical Findings

- Esotropia
- Reduced stereopsis with visual deprivation
- Conjunctival scarring if previous strabismus surgery
- Oblique muscle over-action and dissociated vertical deviation common
- Diplopia may be present

Ancillary Testing

- Cover testing
- Hirschberg or Krimsky light reflex test if unable to perform cover test
- Retinoscopy
- Full ophthalmic examination including slit lamp and fundus

Differential Diagnosis

- Pseudoesotropia
- Congenital esotropia
- Accommodative esotropia
- High AC:A ratio esotropia
- Divergence insufficiency
- Spasm of near reflex
- **Non-comitant strabismus, i.e.:**
  - Duane syndrome type 1 • sixth nerve palsy • ocular myasthenia gravis
    - progressive external ophthalmoplegia • restrictive strabismus

Treatment

- Fully correct cycloplegic refractive error
- Occlusion therapy if amblyopia present
- Bilateral or unilateral medial rectus recession or lateral rectus advancement
- Consider adjustable suture techniques
- **Can treat diplopia with:**
  - occlusion patch • Bangerter foil • prisms

Prognosis

- Ability to restore visual acuity, stereopsis, and ocular alignment depends on underlying cause of consecutive esotropia
- Future surgery may be required for consecutive exotropia or recurrent esotropia if visual acuity and binocular fusion cannot be restored

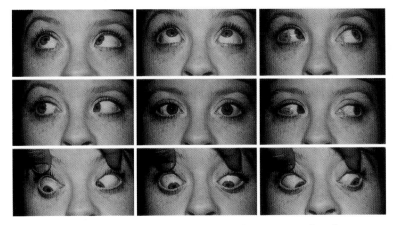

Fig. 10.7 Consecutive esotropia after bilateral lateral rectus recessions for intermittent exotropia.

Deprivation Esotropia

Key Facts

- **Alternative name:** sensory deprivation esotropia
- Constant esotropia secondary to severely reduced vision in one or both eyes
- Typically comitant but can become incomitant over time secondary to contracted medial rectus

Clinical Findings

- Anisometropic amblyopia
- **Organic causes of:**
  - visual deprivation • corneal scarring • cataract • retinal lesions • optic atrophy

Ancillary Testing

- Cycloplegic retinoscopy to determine if anisometropia
- Cover–uncover and alternate cover testing
- Hirschberg or Krimsky light reflex test if unable to perform cover test
- Forced duction testing to determine if medial rectus is contracted

Differential Diagnosis

- Pseudoesotropia
- Congenital esotropia
- Accommodative esotropia
- High AC : A ratio esotropia
- Divergence insufficiency
- Spasm of near reflex
- Consecutive esotropia
- **Non-comitant strabismus, i.e.:**
  - Duane syndrome type 1 • sixth nerve palsy • ocular myasthenia gravis • progressive external ophthalmoplegia • restrictive strabismus

Treatment

- Treat underlying amblyopia or organic lesion if possible during critical period (<6–8 years of age)
- Surgically correct esotropia, monocular recess–resect of visually impaired eye
- Polycarbonate protective lenses to protect seeing eye

Prognosis

- Potential for improved function if treatable underlying cause

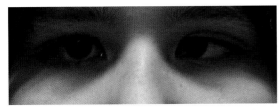

Fig. 10.8 Left deprivation esotropia secondary to aphakia from congenital cataract excision and poor compliance with aphakic contact lens and amblyopia treatment. Visual acuity: counting fingers.

Sixth Nerve Palsy

Key Facts

- Incomitant esotropia secondary to abnormality of sixth nerve, causing lateral rectus muscle dysfunction
- Unilateral or bilateral
- **Causes include:**
  - intracranial mass • increased intracranial pressure • infectious or inflammatory processes • head trauma • microvascular insult

Clinical Findings

- Esotropia worse at distance than near
- Abduction deficit
- Incomitant deviation where esotropia is worse when looking to side of sixth nerve paralysis
- Diplopia in primary position that improves when looking to side opposite sixth nerve paralysis
- May show head turn to side of sixth nerve paralysis to alleviate diplopia
- Negative force ductions with reduced or absent force generations

Ancillary Testing

- Cover–uncover and alternate cover testing at both distance and near
- Maddox rod, Hirschberg, or Krimsky light reflex test if unable to perform cover test
- Force duction or generation testing
- MRI or CT scan with contrast
- Medical and neurologic evaluation
- Consider edrophonium (Tensilon) test

Differential Diagnosis

- Pseudoesotropia
- Congenital esotropia
- Accommodative esotropia
- High AC : A ratio esotropia
- Divergence insufficiency
- Consecutive esotropia
- Deprivation esotropia
- **Non-comitant strabismus, i.e.:**
  - Duane syndrome type 1 • sixth nerve palsy • ocular myasthenia gravis • progressive external ophthalmoplegia • restrictive strabismus

Treatment

- Treat underlying medical or neurologic condition
- Prisms to alleviate diplopia in primary position
- Treat amblyopia
- Consider botulinum into medial rectus muscle antagonist
- Strabismus surgery may be required
  - Horizontal surgery if some lateral rectus function
  - Transposition surgery if limited or no lateral rectus function

Prognosis

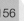

- Depends on underlying medical or neurologic process
- Most vasculopathic and traumatic palsies improve over time

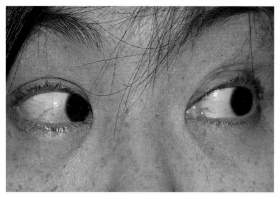

Fig. 10.9 Partial right sixth nerve palsy left gaze. Note full right eye adduction and left eye abduction.

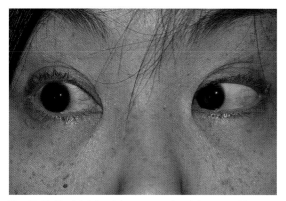

Fig. 10.10 Partial right sixth nerve palsy right gaze. Note limitation of right eye abduction and full left eye adduction.

Duane Syndrome

Key Facts

- **Alternative name:** Duane retraction syndrome
- Congenital hypoplasia or absence of cranial sixth nerve or nucleus
- Abnormal innervation of lateral rectus by third nerve
- 15% bilateral
- More common in women than in men
- Left side more frequently involved
- Face may be turned to affected side
- Vision typically normal
- **Type 1:** limited or absent abduction with relatively normal adduction, esotropic abduction more limited than adduction, esotropic in primary position
- **Type 2:** limited or absent adduction with relative normal abduction, exotropic adduction more limited than abduction, extropic in primary position
- **Type 2:** limited adduction and abduction, orthotropic equal limitation of abduction and adduction, orthotropic in primary position

Clinical Findings

- Limitation or absence of abduction
- Variable limitation of adduction
- Globe retraction and palpebral fissure narrowing on adduction
- Up–down shoot may be present on adduction
- Binocular vision present with face turn

Ancillary Testing

- Cover testing
- Hirschberg or Krimsky light reflex test if unable to perform cover test

Differential Diagnosis

- Congenital esotropia
- Accommodative esotropia
- High AC:A ratio esotropia
- Divergence insufficiency
- Spasm of near reflex
- Consecutive esotropia
- **Non-comitant strabismus, i.e.:**
  - sixth nerve palsy • ocular myasthenia gravis • progressive external ophthalmoplegia • restrictive strabismus

Treatment

- Treat refractive error and amblyopia if present
- **Treatment for head turn:**
  - prisms
  - surgery (medial rectus recession, transposition procedure, lateral rectus Y splitting or recession for up–down shoot)

Prognosis

- Excellent visual prognosis
- Depends on degree of head turn and up–down shoot

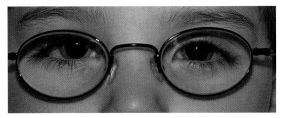

Fig. 10.11 Duane syndrome primary position: orthotropia.

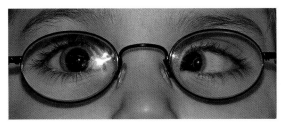

Fig. 10.12 Duane syndrome in right eye. Note limitation of abduction on right gaze with widening of palpebral fissure.

Section

11

Strabismus:
Exodeviations

Pseudoexotropia

Key Facts

- With visual axis aligned, there is a false appearance of exotropia

Clinical Findings

- Wide interpupillary distance
- Positive angle kappa with or without ocular abnormalities, i.e. temporal macular dragging in retinopathy of prematurity
- No movement on cover–uncover test

Ancillary Testing

- Cover testing
- Hirschberg or Krimsky light reflex test if unable to perform cover test
- Full ophthalmic examination including slit lamp and fundus

Differential Diagnosis

- Intermittent exotropia
- Congenital exotropia
- Deprivation exotropia
- Consecutive exotropia
- Convergence insufficiency exotropia
- Convergence paralysis
- **Non-comitant strabismus, i.e.:**
  - Duane syndrome type 2 • partial third nerve palsy • ocular myasthenia gravis • progressive external ophthalmoplegia • restrictive strabismus

Treatment

- None required

Prognosis

- Excellent if no organic lesion discovered causing angle kappa

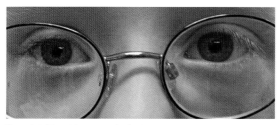

Fig. 11.1 Pseudoexotropia in right eye secondary to positive angle kappa in dragged macula from retinopathy of prematurity.

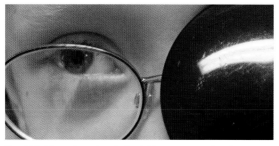

Fig. 11.2 Pseudoexotropia in right eye secondary to positive angle kappa, right eye fixating.

Intermittent Exotropia

Key Facts

- Most common form of divergent strabismus
- Begins in childhood but often decompensates with age
- Amblyopia uncommon unless deviation becomes more frequent
- When eye deviates, stereopsis is lost
- Rare complaint of diplopia when eye drifts
- Deviation worsens when tired, sick, or at times of inattention or intoxication
- Sometimes children close one eye with glare or bright lights

Clinical Findings

- Basic-type exotropia when deviation is similar at both distance and near
- Divergence-type exotropia when deviation is greater at distance than near
- Simulated divergence excess–type exotropia when deviation initially is greater at distance than near but equalized with +3.00 D lens at near or prolonged monocular occlusion
- Convergence insufficiency type when deviation is worse at near than distance
- Mild type when eye easily realigned after cover testing
- Moderate type when eye realigned with blink or eye closure after cover testing
- Severe type when eye realignment prolonged after cover testing

Ancillary Testing

- Cover testing with +3.00 D lens at near or prolonged monocular occlusion may uncover full amount of distance and near deviation
- Hirschberg or Krimsky light reflex test if unable to perform cover test
- Stereopsis testing

Differential Diagnosis

- Pseudoexotropia
- Congenital exotropia
- Deprivational exotropia
- Convergence insufficiency exotropia
- **Non-comitant strabismus, i.e.:**
  - Duane syndrome type 3 • wall-eyed bilateral internuclear ophthalmoplegia (WEBINO) • third nerve palsy • progressive external ophthalmoplegia • ocular myasthesia gravis • restrictive strabismus

Treatment

- Fully correct refractive error
- Stimulate accommodative convergence by prescribing more myopic correction, typically 1 D (under plus or over minus)
- Orthoptic exercises for convergence insufficiency type
- Occlusion therapy if amblyopia present
- Bilateral lateral rectus recessions or uniocular medial rectus resection with lateral rectus recession

Prognosis

- With appropriate treatment in amblyogenic age range, potential for normal acuity and stereopsis is excellent

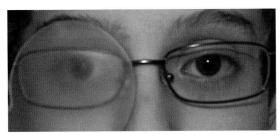

Fig. 11.3 Intermittent right exotropia manifest when eye dissociated under an opaque occluder.

Congenital Exotropia

Key Facts

- Large angle divergent strabismus present at birth or within first year of life
- Associated with neurologic abnormalities or craniofacial syndromes

Clinical Findings

- Exotropia usually >35 PD
- Typically no significant refractive error
- Alternate fixation
- Deviation similar both distance and near

Ancillary Testing

- Cover testing
- Hirschberg or Krimsky light reflex test if unable to perform cover test
- Stereopsis testing
- Consider neurologic referral and neuroimaging if other neurodevelopment abnormalities present

Differential Diagnosis

- Pseudoexotropia
- Intermittent exotropia
- Deprivational exotropia
- Convergence insufficiency exotropia
- **Non-comitant strabismus, i.e.:**
  - Duane syndrome type 3 • wall-eyed bilateral internuclear ophthalmoplegia (WEBINO) • third nerve palsy • progressive external ophthalmoplegia • ocular myasthesia gravis • restrictive strabismus

Treatment

- Fully correct refractive error
- Occlusion therapy if amblyopia present
- Bilateral lateral rectus recessions or monocular medial rectus resection with lateral rectus recession
- With large angles >50 PD, may require surgery on three or four muscles

Prognosis

- If alternate fixation present, visual acuity potential is good
- Despite surgical realignment, development of steropsis is problematic and risk of further surgery or consecutive deviations high

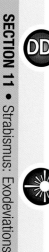

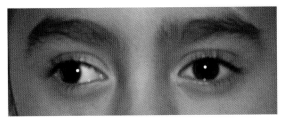

Fig. 11.4 Congenital exotropia, left eye fixating.

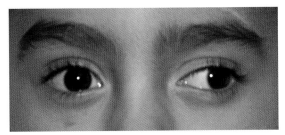

Fig. 11.5 Congenital exotropia, right eye fixating.

Deprivation Exotropia

Key Facts

- Large angle divergent strabismus after reduced acuity in one or both eyes
- Can occur weeks to years after visual loss or with discovery of reduced vision
- Psychosocial dysfunction is an essential aspect of ocular misalignment

Clinical Findings

- Typically large angle exotropia
- Adduction deficits common secondary to lateral rectus contracture
- Oblique muscle over-action and dissociated vertical deviation common
- Diplopia may be present
- **Reduced acuity, common causes including:**
  - ocular trauma • amblyopia • corneal abnormalities (e.g. scars or other opacities) • cataract • retinal diseases • optic nerve hypoplasia or atrophy

Ancillary Testing

- Cover testing
- Hirschberg or Krimsky light reflex test if unable to perform cover test
- Retinoscopy
- Full ophthalmic examination including slit lamp and fundus
- Forced ductions to determine lateral rectus contracture

Differential Diagnosis

- Pseudoexotropia
- Congenital exotropia
- Intermittent exotropia
- Convergence insufficiency exotropia
- **Non-comitant strabismus, i.e.:**
  - Duane syndrome type 3 • wall-eyed bilateral internuclear ophthalmoplegia (WEBINO) • third nerve palsy • ocular myasthenia gravis • progressive external ophthalmoplegia • restrictive strabismus

Treatment

- Fully correct refractive error
- Patch if amblyopia present
- Treat underlying ocular disorder if able
- Bilateral lateral rectus recessions or uniocular medial rectus resection with lateral rectus recession
- **Can treat diplopia with:**
  - occlusion patch • Bangerter foil • prisms
- Protective polycarbonate spectacles

Prognosis

- If acuity restored, diplopia may occur
- Ability to restore visual acuity, stereopsis, and ocular alignment depends on underlying cause of visual loss
- Further surgery may be required in future for consecutive esotropia or recurrent exotropia if visual acuity and fusion cannot be restored

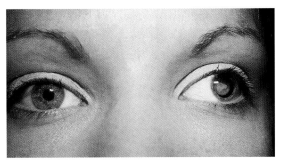

Fig. 11.6 Left deprivation exotropia secondary to a cataract. (From Taylor D, Hoyt CS 2005 Pediatric Ophthalmology and Strabismus, 3rd edn. Saunders, London.)

Consecutive Exotropia

Key Facts

- Divergent strabismus after treatment of esotropia
- Exotropia from slipped or stretched muscle after esotropia surgery
- Exotropia from inability to establish fusion after surgical alignment of esotropia
- Inappropriate surgical alignment of accommodative esotropia now requiring optical correction
- Can occur acutely or years later
- Diplopia may be present and reduced stereopsis

Clinical Findings

- Exotropia
- Reduced stereopsis with visual deprivation
- Conjunctival scarring if past strabismus surgery
- Oblique muscle over-action and dissociated vertical deviation common
- Diplopia may be present
- Hyperopia if accommodative component

Ancillary Testing

- Cover testing
- Hirschberg or Krimsky light reflex test if unable to perform cover test
- Cycloplegic retinoscopy
- Full ophthalmic examination including slit lamp and fundus

Differential Diagnosis

- Pseudoexotropia
- Congenital exotropia
- Intermittent exotropia
- Convergence insufficiency exotropia
- **Non-comitant strabismus, i.e.:**
  - Duane syndrome type 3 • wall-eyed bilateral internuclear ophthalmoplegia (WEBINO) • third nerve palsy • ocular myasthenia gravis • progressive external ophthalmoplegia • restrictive strabismus

Treatment

- Fully correct refractive error
- Occlusion therapy if amblyopia present
- Treat underlying ocular disorder, if able
- Bilateral lateral rectus recession or medial rectus advancement
- Consider adjustable suture techniques
- **Can treat diplopia with:**
  - occlusion patch • Bangerter foil • prisms
- Protective polycarbonate spectacles

Prognosis

- Ability to restore visual acuity, stereopsis, and ocular alignment depends on underlying cause
- Further surgery may be required in future for consecutive esotropia or recurrent exotropia if visual acuity and fusion cannot be restored

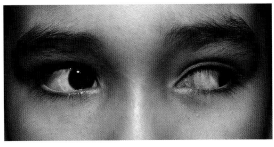

Fig. 11.7 Consecutive exotropia after bilateral medial rectus recessions. Note scar of conjunctiva in region of left medial rectus muscle.

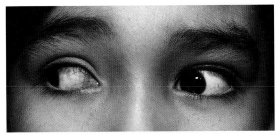

Fig. 11.8 Consecutive exotropia after bilateral medial rectus recessions. Note scar of conjunctiva in region of right medial rectus muscle.

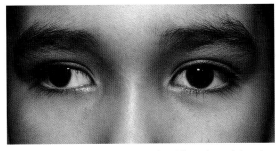

Fig. 11.9 Consecutive exotropia after bilateral medial rectus recessions, primary position.

Convergence Insufficiency

Key Facts

- Exophoria at near secondary to poor convergence
- Worse with prolonged reading, fatigue, or illness
- **Symptoms include:**
  - asthenopia • diplopia • blurry vision • headaches
- May be exacerbated by head trauma or underlying neurologic disease (parkinsonism)

Clinical Findings

- Exophoria at near with minimal or no distance deviation
- Remote near point of convergence

Ancillary Testing

- Cover testing
- Hirschberg or Krimsky light reflex test if unable to perform cover test
- Stereopsis testing
- Consider neurologic referral and neuroimaging if other focal neurologic signs

Differential Diagnosis

- Pseudoexotropia
- Congenital exotropia
- Intermittent exotropia
- Deprivational exotropia
- Convergence paralysis
- **Non-comitant strabismus, i.e.:**
  - Duane syndrome type 3 • wall-eyed bilateral internuclear ophthalmoplegia (WEBINO) • third nerve palsy • progressive external ophthalmoplegia • ocular myasthesia gravis • restrictive strabismus

Treatment

- Correct cycloplegic refractive error
- Orthopic exercises
- Base in prisms in reading glasses
- May require strabismus surgery, but risk of diplopia at distance; medial rectus resections
- Limit extent of prolonged reading, if possible

Prognosis

- **Better prognosis if:**
  - less symptomatic • minimal deviation • response to orthoptic exercises
- Less success for complete improvement if surgery necessary

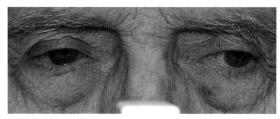

Fig. 11.10 Convergence insufficiency in a patient with Parkinsonism; note near target.

Convergence Paralysis

Key Facts
- Acute onset exotropia and diplopia at near
- Usually secondary to intracranial lesion involving third nerve surround or convergence center
- Associated with Parinaud syndrome

Clinical Findings
- Exotropia on attempted near fixation
- Normal adduction on duction testing

Ancillary Testing
- Cover testing
- Maddox rod, Hirschberg, or Krimsky light reflex test if unable to perform cover test
- MRI scan preferred, or CT with neurologic referral

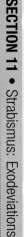

Differential Diagnosis
- Pseudoexotropia
- Congenital exotropia
- Intermittent exotropia
- Deprivational exotropia
- Consecutive exotropia
- Convergence insufficiency exotropia
- **Non-comitant strabismus, i.e.:**
  - Duane syndrome type 3 • wall-eyed bilateral internuclear ophthalmoplegia (WEBINO) • third nerve palsy • progressive external ophthalmoplegia • ocular myasthesia gravis • restrictive strabismus

Treatment
- Correct refractive error
- Base in prisms in reading glasses
- Monocular occlusion

Prognosis
- Depends on response to treatment of underlying neurologic condition

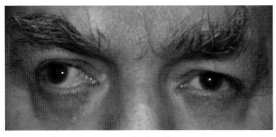

Fig. 11.11 Convergence paralysis, distance.

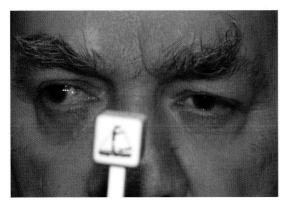

Fig. 11.12 Convergence paralysis, near.

Section

12

Strabismus: Deviations

Inferior Oblique Over-action

Key Facts
- **Associated with:**
  - congenital horizontal strabismus • latent nystagmus • dissociated vertical deviation
- Primary type: over-action commonly develops in patients with congenital esotropia
- Secondary type: over-action due to under-action of antagonist superior oblique muscle in fourth nerve palsy
- Usually bilateral, although typically asymmetric
- May develop head tilt if secondary to superior oblique palsy

Clinical Findings
- Over-elevation on adduction
- Abducted eye hypotropic on alternate cover testing
- V-pattern strabismus
- Positive head tilt test and fundus excyclotorsion with superior oblique palsy

Ancillary Testing
- Cover testing
- Hirschberg or Krimsky light reflex test if unable to perform cover test
- **CT or MRI scan with contract and neurologic referral if:**
  - diplopia • low vertical fusional amplitudes • associated superior oblique palsy

Differential Diagnosis
- Dissociated vertical deviation
- **Non-comitant strabismus, i.e.:**
  - Duane syndrome • ocular myasthenia gravis • progressive external ophthalmoplegia • restrictive strabismus

Treatment
- Fully correct refractive error and treat amblyopia if present
- **Observation if:**
  - good alignment in primary position • no significant V pattern • acceptable appearance
- **Intervention if:**
  - prism: • small deviation • inferior oblique surgery: • recession • anterior transposition • myectomy
- **Inferior oblique surgery:**
  - recession • anterior transposition • myectomy

Prognosis
- Excellent response to surgical intervention if primary type
- Secondary type may require multiple surgeries on other vertical muscles

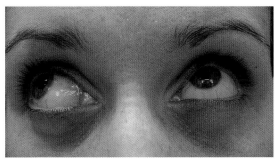
Fig. 12.1 Left inferior oblique over-action.

Inferior Oblique Over-action

Inferior Oblique Palsy

Key Facts

- Rare and controversial entity
- Unknown cause
- Can be confused with Brown syndrome

Clinical Findings

- Elevation deficit in adduction
- A pattern
- May develop head tilt to side of involved eye
- Superior oblique over-action usually present
- Negative force ductions

Ancillary Testing

- Cover testing
- Hirschberg or Krimsky light reflex test if unable to perform cover test
- Force duction testing
- MRI scan with gadolinium and neurologic referral if other focal neurologic signs

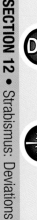

Differential Diagnosis

- Brown syndrome
- Double elevator palsy
- **Non-comitant strabismus, i.e.:**
  - Duane syndrome • ocular myasthenia gravis • progressive external ophthalmoplegia • restrictive strabismus

Treatment

- Fully correct refractive error and treat amblyopia if present
- **Observation if:**
  - good alignment in primary position • no significant A pattern • acceptable appearance
- **Treatment if abnormal head position, diplopia, and significant hypotropia:**
  - prisms • ipsilateral superior oblique weakening • contralateral superior rectus recession

Prognosis

- Visual acuity, stereopsis, and ocular alignment depend on degree of hypotropia, head tilt, and response to treatments, if required
- Risk of torsional diplopia and iatrogenic superior oblique palsy if normal stereopsis and surgery performed on superior oblique muscle
- With small or no head tilt and development of binocular fusion, visual prognosis is excellent

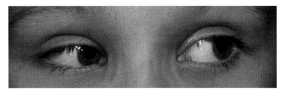

Fig. 12.2 Right inferior oblique palsy.

Superior Oblique Over-action

Key Facts

- Associated with congenital horizontal strabismus, typically exotropia
- Usually bilateral, although typically asymmetric

Clinical Findings

- Over-depression on adduction
- Abducted eye is hypertropic on alternate cover testing
- A-pattern strabismus

Ancillary Testing

- Cover testing
- Hirschberg or Krimsky light reflex test if unable to perform cover test

Differential Diagnosis

- Inferior oblique palsy
- **Non-comitant strabismus, i.e.:**
  - Duane syndrome • ocular myasthenia gravis • progressive external ophthalmoplegia • restrictive strabismus

Treatment

- Fully correct refractive error and treat amblyopia if present
- **Observation if:**
  - good alignment in primary position • no significant A pattern • acceptable appearance
- **Superior oblique surgery:**
  - tenotomy • tendon lengthening with silicone expander or non-absorbable suture

Prognosis

- If surgery is performed on a patient with normal stereopsis, there is a risk of torsional diplopia

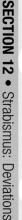

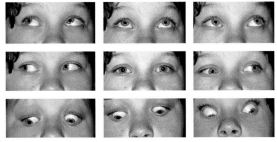

Fig. 12.3 Superior oblique over-action in A-pattern exotropia. (From Taylor D, Hoyt CS 2005 Pediatric Ophthalmology and Strabismus, 3rd edn. Saunders, London.)

Superior Oblique Palsy

Key Facts

- **Alternative name:** fourth or trochlear nerve palsy
- Congenital or acquired
- **Acquired causes:**
  - head trauma • intracranial tumor • vasculopathic (diabetes, hypertension)
- Unilateral or bilateral

Clinical Findings

- Hypertropia in primary position
- Under-depression on adduction
- Over-elevation on adduction if concomitant inferior oblique over-action
- Head tilt to shoulder opposite side of paresis
- Abducted eye hypotropic on alternate cover testing
- V-pattern esotropia and chin depression if bilateral
- Fundus excyclotorsion
- Positive three-step test
- Depression deficit on abduction if ipsilateral superior rectus contraction also present
- Amblyopia may be present

Ancillary Testing

- Cover testing
- Hirschberg or Krimsky light reflex test if unable to perform cover test
- Examine old photographs for head tilt
- Three-step test
- Maddox rod test for excyclotorsion
  - Usually >10° if bilateral
- CT or MRI scan with contract and neurologic referral if diplopia and low vertical fusional amplitudes

Differential Diagnosis

- Dissociated vertical deviation
- Primary inferior oblique over-action
- **Non-comitant strabismus, i.e.:**
  - Duane syndrome • ocular myasthenia gravis • progressive external ophthalmoplegia • restrictive strabismus

Treatment

- Fully correct refractive error and treat amblyopia if present
- **Observation if:**
  - good alignment in primary position • no significant V pattern or head tilt
    - acceptable appearance
- Prism if small deviation and hypertropia in primary position
- **Inferior oblique surgery:**
  - recession • anterior transposition • myectomy
- **Superior oblique surgery:**
  - graded tuck • Harada–Ito for torsion
- Contralateral inferior recession
- Ipsilateral superior rectus recession

Prognosis

- Risk of iatrogenic Brown syndrome if superior oblique tuck performed
- May require multiple surgeries. If vasculopathic or traumatic high-rate spontaneous improvement

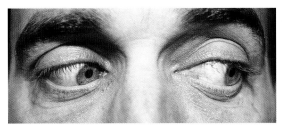

Fig. 12.4 Left superior oblique palsy, left down gaze.

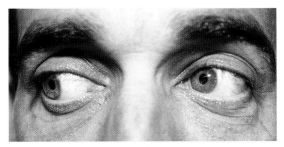

Fig. 12.5 Left superior oblique palsy, right down gaze.
Note under-action in region of left superior oblique.

Dissociated Vertical Deviation

Key Facts

- Commonly found in patients who do not develop binocularity
- Associated with congenital horizontal strabismus and latent nystagmus
- Occurs when eye is occluded or during visual inattention
- Usually bilateral, although typically asymmetric

Clinical Findings

- Eye drifts upward and outward and excyclotorts
- No upward movement of fixating eye, as upward deviating eye moves down to fixate

Ancillary Testing

- Cover testing
- Hirschberg or Krimsky light reflex test if unable to perform cover test
- Retinoscopy
- Full ophthalmic examination including slit lamp and fundus

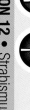

Differential Diagnosis

- Over-acting inferior oblique muscle
- Hypertropia from nerve paresis, restrictive strabismus, or ocular myasthenia

Treatment

- Fully correct refractive error if present
- Patch if amblyopia present
- **Surgical correction:**
  - superior rectus recession with or without posterior fixation suture (Faden)
    - inferior oblique anterior transposition • inferior rectus resection

Prognosis

- Ability to restore visual acuity, stereopsis, and ocular alignment depends on underlying cause
- Future surgery may be required for consecutive esotropia or recurrent exotropia if visual acuity and binocular fusion cannot be restored

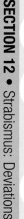

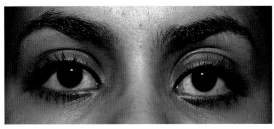

Fig. 12.6 Dissociated vertical deviation in right eye with left eye fixating.

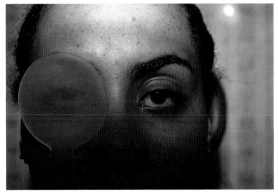

Fig. 12.7 Dissociated vertical deviation, left eye fixating.

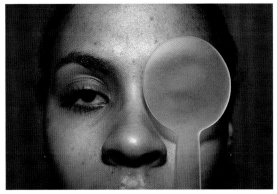

Fig. 12.8 Dissociated vertical deviation, right eye fixating.

Brown Syndrome

Key Facts

- Deficient elevation on adduction secondary to restriction of superior oblique tendon at trochlear pulley
- May be bilateral and congenital
- May be acquired and appear suddenly and resolve spontaneously
- May have diplopia that resolves with chin-up posture or amblyopia
- **Association with:**
  - trochlea trauma • inflammatory diseases • sinusitis

Clinical Findings

- Deficient elevation on adduction
- Improved elevation on abduction
- Divergence can occur with midline elevation; V pattern
- May be hypotropic in primary position
- Positive force ductions

Ancillary Testing

- Cover testing
- Hirschberg or Krimsky light reflex test if unable to perform cover test
- Retinoscopy
- Full ophthalmic examination including slit lamp and fundus
- Force duction testing

Differential Diagnosis

- Hypotropia from nerve paresis, restrictive strabismus, or ocular myasthenia gravis

Treatment

- Fully correct refractive error if present
- Patch if amblyopia present
- Treat systemic condition with non-steroidal anti-inflammatory agents or corticosteroids
- Corticosteroid injection in region of trochlea
- **Surgical correction:**
  - ipsilateral superior oblique tenotomy with or without ipsilateral inferior oblique weakening
  - graded recession using superior oblique tendon spacer

Prognosis

- Depends on degree of hypotropia in primary position leading to amblyopia, loss of steropsis, or diplopia

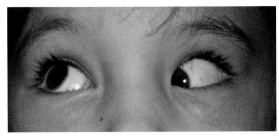
Fig. 12.9 Brown syndrome in left eye.

Double-elevator Palsy
(Monocular Elevator Palsy)

Key Facts

- Deficit of elevation in all fields of gaze
- Weakness of superior rectus and inferior oblique muscles or deficit innervations
- Bell phenomenon present if supranuclear cause
- Concomitant ipsilateral inferior rectus restriction

Clinical Findings

- Limitation of elevation in primary position, adduction, and abduction
- May have chin elevation to maintain fusion
- Amblyopia of hypotropic eye may be present
- Ptosis may be present when fixating with uninvolved eye
- Secondary hypertropia of unaffected eye when fixating with affected eye

Ancillary Testing

- Cover testing
- Hirschberg or Krimsky light reflex test if unable to perform cover test
- Retinoscopy
- Full ophthalmic examination including slit lamp and fundus
- Force duction testing
- Consider MRI scan with gadolinium

Differential Diagnosis

- Brown syndrome
- Ocular myasthenia gravis, progressive external ophthalmoplegia, or restrictive strabismus

Treatment

- Fully correct refractive error if present
- Patch if amblyopia present
- **Surgical correction, chin elevation, and/or large hypotropia in primary position:**
    - inferior rectus recession if restriction present
    - transposition of medial and lateral rectus to insertion of superior rectus
    - may require subsequent ptosis repair
    - Inferior rectus recession may be required if diplopia or hypotropia in primary position

Prognosis

- Visual acuity, stereopsis, and ocular alignment depend on degree of hypotropia, chin elevation, and response to treatments if required
- With small or no chin elevation and development of fusion, visual prognosis is excellent

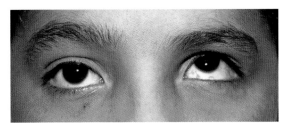

Fig. 12.10 Double elevator palsy in right eye.

Orbital Floor Fracture

Key Facts

- Limited vertical gaze secondary to entrapment of or injury to inferior rectus or inferior oblique muscle
- Typically occurs when object larger than the globe impacts orbital rim
- High association with other orbit fractures, most notably the medial wall, leading to horizontal gaze deficits
- If inferior rectus is entrapped within the fracture, this can lead to limited elevation and hypotropia of the involved eye that worsens on up gaze
- If nerve supply to inferior rectus is involved or a posterior fracture is present, a relative hypertropia of the involved eye with a depression deficit that is worse on down gaze may result

Clinical Findings

- Diplopia with limited vertical extraocular movements
- Ecchymosis
- Tissue crepitus due to sinus air entrapment within surrounding soft tissues
- Enophthalmus depends on extent of fracture
- Possible paresthesia or hypoesthesia secondary to damage of infraorbital nerve
- Possible associated globe or optic nerve injury

Ancillary Testing

- Full ophthalmic examination including visual acuity assessment and cover–uncover test
- Trigeminal distribution sensory testing
- Force ductions to determine if restrictive versus paretic
- CT scan of orbits with direct axial and coronal views
- MRI scan of orbit with gadolinium, fat saturation sequences

Differential Diagnosis

- Cranial nerve palsy
- **Non-comitant strabismus, i.e.:**
  - Duane syndrome • ocular myasthenia gravis • progressive external ophthalmoplegia • restrictive strabismus

Treatment

- Appropriate treatment of related globe or optic nerve injury if present
- Antibiotic prophylaxis to prevent orbital cellulitis
- Prisms or optical occlusion to eliminate diplopia
- Repair of fracture if risk for enophthalmos or persistent diplopia (larger fracture with displacement of orbital contents)

Prognosis

- Depends on extent of fracture, muscle, and if any associated globe injury
- Even despite repair, diplopia my persist, necessitating prisms or extraocular muscle surgery

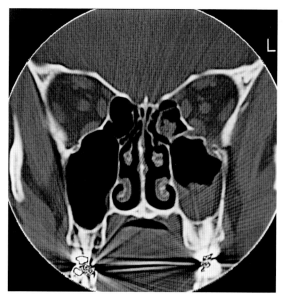

Fig. 12.11 Coronal CT showing left orbital floor fracture with entrapment of left inferior rectus muscle.

Section

13

Strabismus: Miscellaneous

Thyroid Orbitopathy

Key Facts

- Restrictive myopathy secondary to thyroid-associated autoimmune disease
- Lymphocyte infiltration leading to inflammation, edema, and fibrosis of orbital tissues including extraocular muscles
- Rare in children, especially before puberty
- Can be euthyroid, hypothyroid, or hyperthyroid
- Smoking aggravates myopathy
- Variable diplopia
- Association with ocular myasthenia gravis

Clinical Findings

- Restrictive motility, force duction positive
- Hypotropia and esotropia most common
- Proptosis
- Possible compressive optic neuropathy
- Possible elevated IOP

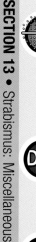

Ancillary Testing

- Cover testing
- Hirschberg or Krimsky light reflex test if unable to perform cover test
- Force duction testing
- Color vision testing
- Exophthalmometry
- Consider CT or MRI with contrast of orbits, tendon sparing muscle enlargement
- Consider testing for ocular myasthenia gravis

Differential Diagnosis

- Third nerve palsy
- Sixth nerve palsy
- **Other non-comitant strabismus, i.e.:**
  - Duane syndrome • ocular myasthenia gravis • progressive external ophthalmoplegia • orbital fracture

Treatment

- Corticosteroids or orbital irradiation if significant inflammatory component, although controversial
- Prisms for small deviation in primary position
- **Extraocular muscle surgery for correction of larger deviations in primary position:**
  - hang-back recession using adjustable techniques
- Orbital decompression if compressive optic neuropathy

Prognosis

- Despite extraocular muscle surgery, typically persistent diplopia on extreme gazes
- Smoking risk factor for severe orbitopathy

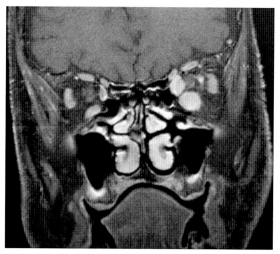

Fig. 13.1 Coronal fat saturation MRI with gadolinium, showing thickening of left medial and inferior rectus in thyroid orbitopathy.

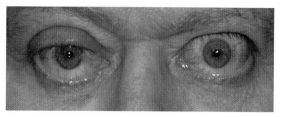

Fig. 13.2 Bilateral proptosis and lid retraction in thyroid orbitopathy. Right ptosis suggests concomittant myasthesia gravis.

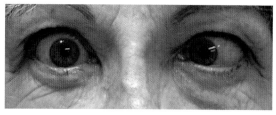

Fig. 13.3 Left extropia and lid retraction in thyroid orbitopathy.

Third Nerve Palsy

Key Facts

- Incomitant exotropia and hypotropia secondary to abnormality of the third nerve, causing dysfunction of medial rectus, superior rectus, inferior rectus, and inferior oblique muscles
- Unilateral or bilateral
- Contralateral superior rectus involvement and bilateral ptosis if third nerve nuclear in origin
- **Causes include:**
  - congenital • intracranial mass • increased intracranial pressure • infectious or inflammatory processes • head trauma • aneurysm

Clinical Findings

- Adduction, elevation, and depression deficit with diplopia
- Ptosis
- Pupil fixed and dilated
- Incomplete palsy and aberrant regeneration can occur
- Negative force ductions with reduced or absent force generations

Ancillary Testing

- Cover–uncover and alternate cover testing at both distance and near
- Hirschberg or Krimsky light reflex test if unable to perform cover test
- Medical and neurologic evaluation
- Force duction or generation testing
- MRI scan with gadolinium contrast
- Magnetic resonance angiography
- Consider edrophonium (Tensilon) test

Differential Diagnosis

- **Non-comitant strabismus, i.e.:**
  - Duane syndrome type 3 • sixth nerve palsy • ocular myasthenia gravis
    - progressive external ophthalmoplegia • restrictive strabismus

Treatment

- Treat underlying medical or neurologic condition
- Prisms to alleviate diplopia in primary position
- Treat amblyopia
- **Strabismus surgery may be required:**
  - horizontal surgery if some medial rectus function
  - superior oblique transposition surgery combined with lateral rectus recession if limited or no medial rectus function

Prognosis

- Depends on underlying medical or neurologic process
- Most vasculopathic and traumatic palsies improve over time
- Difficult to fully correct ocular misalignment

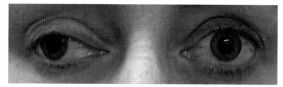

Fig. 13.4 Partial right third nerve palsy showing ptosis and exotropia in primary position.

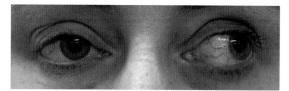

Fig. 13.5 Partial right third nerve palsy showing medial rectus weakness on left gaze.

Myasthenia Gravis

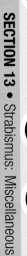

Key Facts

- **Rapid fatigability of:**
  - extraocular muscles • levator • orbicularis oculi
- Purely ocular or generalized
- Impaired neurotransmission secondary to blockage or degradation of acetylcholine receptors
- Associated thymoma

Clinical Findings

- Variable ptosis
- Variable ophthalmoparesis
- Upper eyelid twitching on vertical saccade refixation, Cogan lid twitch

Ancillary Testing

- Cover testing
- Hirschberg or Krimsky light reflex test if unable to perform cover test
- Force duction testing
- Sleep, ice, or edrophonium (Tensilon) test
- Electromyography
- Acetylcholine receptor antibodies
- Chest CT scan
- Neurologic referral

Differential Diagnosis

- **Non-comitant strabismus, i.e.:**
  - Duane syndrome • chronic progressive external ophthalmoplegia • cranial neuropathy • restrictive strabismus

Treatment

- Cholinesterase inhibitors or oral prednisone
- Immunosuppression or thymectomy
- Strabismus repair for stabilized ocular misalignment

Prognosis

- 50% of ocular cases become generalized and may be prevented with early immunosuppression
- Acute malignant form may progress to respiratory failure

Chronic Progressive External Ophthalmoplegia

Key Facts

- Slowly progressive ptosis and ophthalmoparesis
- Mitochondrial myopathy
- Ragged red fibers on muscle biopsy
- Kearns–Sayre syndrome, chronic progressive external ophthalmoplegia (CPEO), pigmentary retinopathy, cardiac conduction defects

Clinical Findings

- Ptosis
- Ophthalmoparesis; exotropia initially
- Diplopia uncommon

Ancillary Testing

- Cover testing
- Hirschberg or Krimsky light reflex test if unable to perform cover test
- Force duction testing
- Electrocardiogram
- Genetics, cardiology, and neurologic referral

Differential Diagnosis

- **Non-comitant strabismus, i.e.:**
  - Duane syndrome • ocular myasthenia gravis • cranial neuropathy • restrictive strabismus

Treatment

- Treatment limited
- Prisms if small deviation in primary position
- Possible ptosis repair
- Strabismus repair typically unsuccessful

Prognosis

- Poor overall prognosis
- Ptosis repair may lead to exposure keratopathy

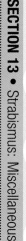

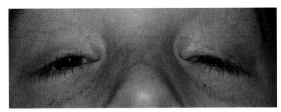

Fig. 13.6 CPEO, primary position.

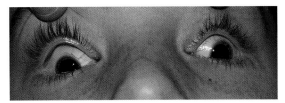

Fig. 13.7 CPEO, attempted left and up gaze.

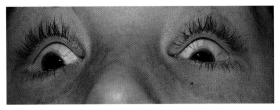

Fig. 13.8 CPEO, attempted right and up gaze.

Congenital Fibrosis

Key Facts

- **Alternative name:** congenital fibrosis of the extraocular muscles (CFEOM)
- Variable fibrosis of otherwise normal extraocular muscle
- **Also includes:**
  - fibrosis of Tenon's capsule
  - globe and Tenon's adhesions to extraocular muscle
  - inelasticity and fragility of conjunctiva
- **CFEOM type 1:**
  - autosomal dominant • bilateral ptosis • aberrant horizontal gaze • eyes fixed in downward position with absent elevation
- **CFEOM type 2:**
  - autosomal recessive • bilateral ptosis • exotropia
- **CFEOM type 3:**
  - autosomal dominant • vertical deficit worse than horizontal deficit
- Caused by aberrant development of midbrain and pontine motor nuclei

Clinical Findings

- Little or no horizontal movement
- Eyes typically fixed 20–30° below horizontal plane
- Blepharoptosis
- Chin elevation
- Amblyopia

Ancillary Testing

- Cover testing
- Hirschberg or Krimsky light reflex test if unable to perform cover test
- Full ophthalmic examination including slit-lamp biomicroscopy and sensory testing
- Force duction testing

Differential Diagnosis

- Infantile esotropia
- Congenital sixth nerve palsy
- Double-elevator palsy
- Möbius syndrome
- **Non-comitant strabismus, i.e.:**
  - Duane syndrome • ocular myasthenia gravis • progressive external ophthalmoplegia • restrictive strabismus

Treatment

- Fully correct refractive error in both eyes with glasses and treat underlying amblyopia
- Strabismus repair to include possible medial rectus recession and vertical rectus muscle transpositions to lateral rectus muscle, utilizing possible adjustable suture techniques
- Ptosis repair
  - Corneal exposure may result

Prognosis

- **Depends on:**
  - extent of ocular misalignment • amblyopia • ptosis • exposure keratopathy

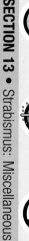

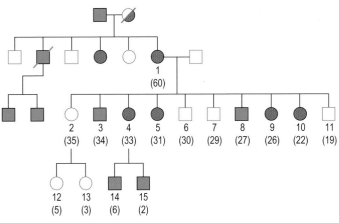

Fig. 13.9 Pedigree of a family with congenital fibrosis syndrome type 1, showing autosomal dominant transmission. (From Taylor D, Hoyt CS 2005 Pediatric Ophthalmology and Strabismus, 3rd edn. Saunders, London.)

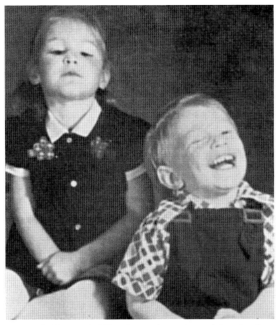

Fig. 13.10 Congenital fibrosis syndrome type 1 in a brother and sister. Because of the bilateral ptosis and deficient upgaze, both children have adopted a head posture with the chin elevated. (Courtesy of Dr Stewart M. Wolff.)

Möbius Syndrome

Key Facts

- Usually bilateral condition affecting brainstem nuclei development of cranial nerves 6, 7, and lower, including paramedian pontine reticular formation
- **Chromosome deletion:** 13q12.2–13
- **Ocular misalignment in association with:**
  - difficulty swallowing and sucking • inability to close eyes • mask-like faces

Clinical Findings

- Sixth nerve palsy with esotropia and inability to abduct
- Seventh nerve palsy with incomplete eyelid closure and mask-like faces
- Exposure keratitis
- Amblyopia may be present
- Absent stereopsis
- May have tongue, limb, and chest abnormalities

Ancillary Testing

- Full ophthalmic examination including slit-lamp biomicroscopy and sensory testing

Differential Diagnosis

- Infantile esotropia
- Duane syndrome
- Congenital sixth nerve palsy
- Oculomotor apraxia

Treatment

- Fully correct refractive error and treat underlying amblyopia
- Strabismus repair to consider medial rectus recession and vertical rectus muscle transpositions to lateral rectus muscle, utilizing possible adjustable suture techniques
- Ocular lubricants or eyelid procedure if significant seventh nerve palsy and exposure keratopathy

Prognosis

- Depends on extent of ocular misalignment, amblyopia, and exposure keratopathy

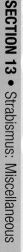

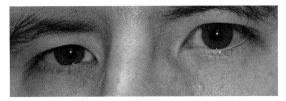

Fig. 13.11 Möbius syndrome.

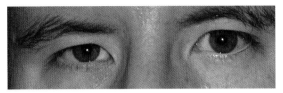

Fig. 13.12 Attempted right gaze.

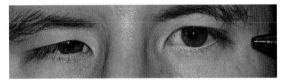

Fig. 13.13 Attempted left gaze.

Möbius Syndrome

Internuclear Ophthalmoplegia

Key Facts

- Lesion involving medial longitudinal fasciculus that connects sixth nerve nucleus to contralateral medial rectus subnucleus
- Separate interneurons that allow for conjugate eye movements
- Bilateral internuclear ophthalmoplegia leads to exotropia in primary position, wall-eyed bilateral internuclear ophthalmoplegia (WEBINO)
- **Most common causes:**
  - demyelinating disease • cerebrovascular accidents • tumors

Clinical Findings

- Adduction limitation or lag
- Contralateral abducting nystagmus
- Convergence typically present
- Variable diplopia

Ancillary Testing

- Cover testing
- Hirschberg or Krimsky light reflex test if unable to perform cover test
- Force duction testing
- MRI with gadolinium and neurologic referral

Differential Diagnosis

- Third nerve palsy
- Exotropia
- **Non-comitant strabismus, i.e.:**
  - Duane syndrome • ocular myasthenia gravis • progressive external ophthalmoplegia • restrictive strabismus

Treatment

- Treat underlying neurologic disorder
- Prisms if small deviation in primary position
- **Strabismus repair:** recess–resect procedure

Prognosis

- Depends on underlying neurologic disorder
- Esotropia at near with resect procedure if convergence present

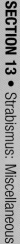

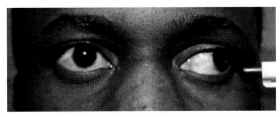

Fig. 13.14 Right internuclear ophthalmoplegia with right
medial rectus weakness on left gaze.

Congenital Ocular Motor Apraxia

Key Facts
- Inability to initiate normal voluntary horizontal saccades
- **Associated with:**
  - developmental delay • hypotonia and intracranial abnormalities • agenesis of corpus callosum • cerebellar vermian hypoplasia

Clinical Findings
- Head-thrusting movements associated with a blink in order to change and maintain fixation
- Preserved vestibular ocular responses

Ancillary Testing
- MRI with gadolinium and neurologic referral

Differential Diagnosis
- Similar findings can be seen in the early stages of leukodystrophy and other metabolic abnormalities that can effect the central nervous system

Treatment
- Treat underlying neurologic or metabolic disorder if present

Prognosis
- Eye movements and head thrusting improves with age
- Depends on underlying neurologic disorder

Section
14
Strabismus: Nystagmus

Congenital Nystagmus

Key Facts

- Slow phase with exponential increase in velocity
- Dampened by convergence, nystagmus blockage syndrome
- Oscillopsia is rare
- Disappears with sleep
- Autosomal dominant, recessive, or X-linked

Clinical Findings

- Binocular conjugate nystagmus
- Usually horizontal and remains so on up and down gaze
- Pendular, jerk, or combination
- Possible esotropia to dampen nystagmus
- Null point or zone may be present with head turn
- Visual acuity may be near normal if null zone present
- Increases with fixation attempt

Ancillary Testing

- Full ophthalmic examination
- Consider electroretinogram to rule out sensory retinal abnormality
- Low vision referral

Differential Diagnosis

- Sensory deficit nystagmus
- Periodic alternating nystagmus
- Latent nystagmus

Treatment

- Correct refractive error and treat amblyopia if present
- Contact lenses
- Prisms to induce convergence dampening
- **Surgery:**
  - correct strabismus
  - correct head position
  - four horizontal muscle retroequatorial recessions or tenotomy with reattachment

Prognosis

- Depends on degree of nystagmus, initial visual acuity, and whether strabismus or abnormal head position develops

---

Box 14.1 Summary of clinical features of congenital nystagmus

Present since infancy
Usually conjugate, horizontal; smaller torsional, or vertical components
Pendular or increasing-velocity waveforms punctuated by foveation periods, during which eyes are transiently still and aimed at the object of interest
Suppresses on convergence or with eyelid closure
Accentuated by visual attention of arousal
Often minimal when the eyes are near one particular orbital position (null zone)
Accompanied by head shaking or head turn

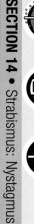

(From Taylor D, Hoyt CS 2005 Pediatric Ophthalmology and Strabismus, 3rd edn. Saunders, London.)

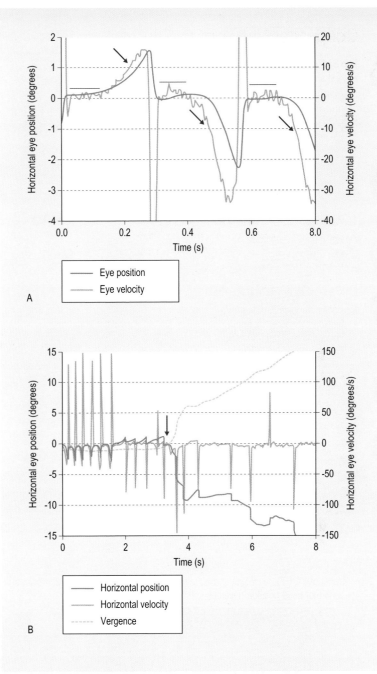

Fig. 14.1 Example of congenital nystagmus. Right eye record. Rightward movements are indicated by upward deflections. (**a**) One rightward followed by two leftward slow phases all show increasing velocity waveforms (arrows). Foveation periods, when the eye is pointed at the target (about zero eye position) and eye velocity is <5°/s, are demarcated by horizontal bars. (**b**) Effects of convergence on nystagmus. After the vertical arrow, the subject started to slowly converge (upward deflections) as she viewed an approaching target aligned on her midline; nystagmus was almost completely suppressed. (From Taylor D, Hoyt CS 2005 Pediatric Ophthalmology and Strabismus, 3rd edn. Saunders, London.)

Spasmus Nutans

Key Facts

- Acquired nystagmus that presents between 3 months and 1 year of age
- **Triad:**
  - nystagmus • head bobbing • torticollis
- Bilateral, asymmetric, and sometimes difficult to see
- May be familial
- Association with chiasmal or suprachiasmal tumors, especially glioma

Clinical Findings

- Dysconjugate small-amplitude, high-frequency oscillations
- Head bobbing
- Strabismus and amblyopia may be present in eye with greatest nystagmus

Ancillary Testing

- MRI with gadolinium

Differential Diagnosis

- Congenital motor nystagmus
- Sensory deficit nystagmus
- Periodic alternating nystagmus
- Latent nystagmus

Treatment

- Correct refractive error and treat amblyopia if present
- Treat intracranial tumor if present

Prognosis

- Usually disappears by age 3 years
- Depends on whether intracranial tumor present

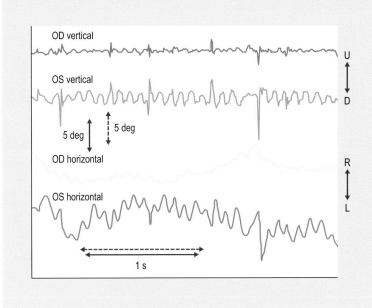

Fig. 14.2 Ocular motility recordings of spasmus nutans. OU open high-frequency (12–14 Hz), asymmetric, dysconjugate, multiplanar, (torsional) pendular nystagmus typical of spasmus nutans. Continuous periods of time are depicted in each tracing. Rightward eye movements are up and leftward eye movements are down. OD, right eye; OS, left eye; OU, both eyes. (From Taylor D, Hoyt CS 2005 Pediatric Ophthalmology and Strabismus, 3rd edn. Saunders, London.)

Index

Index

Index